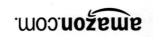

Billing Address:
Alice Daniele
22W281 McCarron Rd.
Glen Ellyn, Illinois 60137
United States

Your order of August 28, 2007 (Order ID 102-7925849-8268925)

Qty.	Item
	IN THIS SHIPMENT
1	**Living and Dying with Dementia: Dialogues about Palliative Care**
	Small, Neil — — Paperback
	(** P-4-M29C27 **) 0198566875
	0198566875

Subtotal
Shipping & Han
Promotional Ce
Order Total
Paid via Discov*
Balance due

This shipment completes your order.

Living and dying with dementia

Living and dying with dementia
Dialogues about palliative care

Neil Small
Professor of Health Research
University of Bradford, UK

Katherine Froggatt
Senior Lecturer, Institute for Health Research
Lancaster University, UK

Murna Downs
Professor of Dementia Studies
University of Bradford, UK

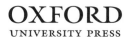
OXFORD
UNIVERSITY PRESS

OXFORD
UNIVERSITY PRESS

Great Clarendon Street, Oxford OX2 6DP

Oxford University Press is a department of the University of Oxford.
It furthers the University's objective of excellence in research, scholarship,
and education by publishing worldwide in

Oxford New York

Auckland Cape Town Dar es Salaam Hong Kong Karachi
Kuala Lumpur Madrid Melbourne Mexico City Nairobi
New Delhi Shanghai Taipei Toronto

With offices in

Argentina Austria Brazil Chile Czech Republic France Greece
Guatemala Hungary Italy Japan Poland Portugal Singapore
South Korea Switzerland Thailand Turkey Ukraine Vietnam

Oxford is a registered trade mark of Oxford University Press
in the UK and in certain other countries

Published in the United States
by Oxford University Press Inc., New York

A catalogue record for this title is available from the British Library
Data available

Library of Congress Cataloging in Publication Data
Small, Neil.
  Living and dying with dementia : dialogues about palliative care / Neil Small,
Katherine Froggatt, Murna Downs.
      p. ; cm.
  Includes bibliographical references and index.
  ISBN 978-0-19-856687-8 (alk. paper)
  1. Dementia–Patients–Care. 2. Dementia–Psychological aspects. 3. Palliative
treatment. I. Froggatt, Katherine. II. Downs, Murna. III. Title.
  [DNLM: 1. Dementia–therapy. 2. Aged. 3. Palliative Care. 4. Patient-Centered
Care. 5. Terminally Ill–psychology. WM 220 S635L 2007]
  RC521.S59 2007
  616.8′3–dc22   2007018599

Typeset by Cepha Imaging Private Ltd., Bangalore, India
Printed in Great Britain
on acid-free paper by
Biddles Ltd., King's Lynn, Norfolk, UK

ISBN 978-0-19-856687-8

10 9 8 7 6 5 4 3 2 1

Whilst every effort has been made to ensure that the contents of this book are as
complete, accurate and up-to-date as possible at the date of writing, Oxford
University Press is not able to give any guarantee or assurance that such is the case.
Readers are urged to take appropriately qualified medical advice in all cases. The
information in this book is intended to be useful to the general reader, but should
not be used as a means of self-diagnosis or for the prescription of medication.

In memory of
Maureen and Tom Downs
and
Alan and Gwen Kidd

You think because you understand one
you must understand *two*,
because one and one makes two.
But you must also understand *and*.

Jelaluddin Rumi, 13th century Sufi saying

Contents

Preface

In those parts of the world where deaths caused by infectious diseases are decreasing and where life expectancy is increasing, a major challenge for the twenty-first century will be the rising incidence and prevalence of chronic illnesses. One of these chronic illnesses is dementia. Inevitably, people living with dementia will die, but the way in which this dying is conceptualized and managed will affect care for the person with dementia, and support for their family. The care of dying people, particularly those with cancer, has been influenced by innovations in palliative care. However, many chronic conditions, including dementia, pose significant challenges for palliative care as it is currently configured.

This book presents the experience of living and dying with dementia, drawing upon narratives of personal experience and examples of care initiatives. The leading specialties that attend to the needs of people with dementia and their families are identified. Each emphasizes different aspects of care and, in so doing, their approaches reflect the underlying values of the specialty.

One of the most innovative approaches to understanding the needs of people with dementia is person-centred care. Strong similarities exist between this and palliative care. Both emphasize the importance of promoting quality of life, and both define quality of life broadly. Both approaches are concerned with the importance of relationships, particularly those with family members and with paid carers. Both are concerned with seeking to access the experience of the person and their family and building care regimes from a process of reconciling these experiences with the resources available. Overall, both person-centred dementia care and palliative care have developed in a way that has combined careful listening to the person and family with learning from innovative practice. However, to date there has been little sharing of the values and experiences between these two approaches. Each has much to contribute, and much to learn, from the other.

This book makes a case for the importance of accessing the subjective experience of living with a life-limiting condition, or of caring for someone with such a condition. It seeks to build an ethic of care from such subjectivities. At the same time it recognizes that people live with dementia and other life-limiting conditions within a particular social context. We explore the interaction of individual experience and social context via a consideration of how the 'journey' of dementia is described by those closest to it. We ask what dementia illustrates in terms of how the self is understood, and we are critical of an assumption that autonomy is central to the self, an assumption that acts contrary to the interests of people with dementia. We explore the way services have developed and consider practice that can emerge from an engagement between the imperatives of the health and social care system and subjectivity. Specifically we do this by focusing on a consideration of how services are constructed to meet particular ideals of quality and on how society manages and positions older people, people with dementia and people who are dying. A point of focus in this book, and a place where many of our concerns are brought together, is our consideration of what a good death with dementia might look like.

The book will be of interest to practitioners in the care of older people, in palliative care and in the care of people with dementia, across a range of care settings. It will be of interest to those concerned with the meaning of care and the social and philosophical understanding of dementia and dying in contemporary society. It will be of relevance to academics and students across a range of disciplines and will address the wider concerns felt by people with dementia and people caring for someone with dementia. We hope it will resonate with their experiences.

Acknowledgements

We are grateful for the generosity of our families and friends who have shared their experiences of living with dementia for this book. Thank you Declan Downs, Deirdre Downs, Ronan Downs, Emer Downs, Alison Kidd and Hugh Kidd.

We are also grateful to Alison Kidd and Hugh Kidd for their careful reading of an earlier draft of this book and for the insightful comments that we hope have improved the version we present now. We are grateful to Dr David Jolley, Dr Shubhra Singh and Professor Dawn Brooker who looked at and commented on parts of the manuscript. Patricia Baldwin helped with proof reading. We want to thank Georgia Pinteau and Clare Caruana at Oxford University Press for their support throughout.

Last but not least we thank Hapé Smeele, who has provided us with his photographs, taken in Holland and Bhutan.

We acknowledge permissions to reproduce the following materials.

From *Watching for the Kingfisher* by Ann Lewin, published by Inspire. Reprinted by permission of the author.

From the Alzheimer's Society newsletters, published by the Alzheimer's Society. Reprinted by permission of the Alzheimer's Society.

From *Alive with Alzheimer's* by Cathy Stein Greenblaat, published by The University of Chicago Press. Reprinted by permission of the author Heather Davidson (heatherelin@yahoo.com).

From *Alzheimer. A Journey Together* by Federica Caracciolo, published by Jessica Kingsley Publishers. Reprinted by permission of Jessica Kingsley Publishers.

From *Openings* by John Killick and Carl Cordonnier, published by Hawker Publications. Reprinted by permission of Hawker Publications and John Killick.

From *The House on Beartown Road* by Elizabeth Cohen, copyright © 2003 by Elizabeth Cohen. Use by permission of The Random House Group Ltd.

From *Have the Men had Enough?* by Margaret Forster. Copyright © 1989, Margaret Foster. By kind permission of the artist and The Sayle Literary Agency.

From *Scar Tissue* by Michael Ignatieff, published by Chatto and Windus. Reprinted by permission of The Random House Group Ltd.

From *The Needs of Strangers* by Michael Ignatieff, copyright © 1985 by Michael Ignatieff. Used by permission of Viking Penguin, a division of Penguin Group (USA) Inc.

From The Assessment by Bernard MacLaverty, published in *New Dubliners* by New Island Books. Reprinted by permission of New Island Books.

From *Untold Stories* by Alan Bennett, published by Faber and Faber. Reproduced by permission from Faber and Faber.

From *Black Daisies for the Bride* by Tony Harrison, published by Faber and Faber. Reproduced by permission from Faber and Faber.

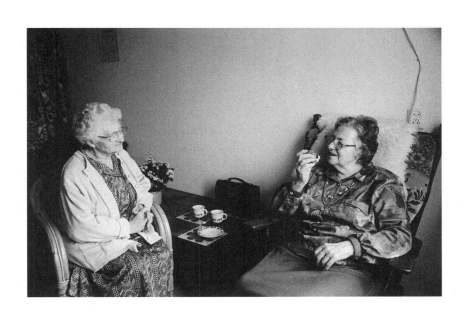

Chapter 1

Introduction

I can remember how when I was young I believed
death to be a phenomenon of the body; now I know it
to be merely a function of the mind – and that of the
minds of the ones who suffer the bereavement. The
nihilists say it is the end; the fundamentalists, the
beginning; when in reality it is no more than a single
tenant or family moving out of a tenement or a town.
Doctor Peabody in (William Faulkner, As I lay dying
1930: 43–4)

It is now recognized that dementia is a terminal condition which, if the person
does not die from some other cause, will lead to an individual's death. Thus while
the person with dementia may not die of dementia they will certainly die *with*
dementia. How long, in what circumstances, and how well a person with dementia lives until they die varies. In focusing on living and dying with dementia in
this book, we will seek to put the person with dementia at the heart of our writing. The person with dementia, like all people, lives within a social network and,
therefore, the experiences of family and friends, members of local communities
and health and social care staff will also be our concern.

The needs that people with dementia have that are associated with their
dying have been neglected. An important cause of this neglect is that people
with dementia have been consigned to the category of the 'already dead'.
This is a category that has a long history. It has been used in relation to leprosy
and to madness (Foucault 1967), it could have been applied to people living
with tuberculosis, cancer or AIDS, indeed it is a category that has included
people living with many serious or life-limiting conditions. Thinking of a
person as already dead explains why only minimal care has been provided
for them, but there are examples of emerging ways of thinking, and alternative structures of practice, that have improved the possibility of living well
until you die, even if you have a 'dread' disease. One such way of thinking is
present in the philosophy and practice of palliative care. We will look at its

contribution to care for dying people and consider, specifically, its potential for people with dementia.

In this chapter, we initially provide an overview of the numbers of people with dementia. We then go on to outline key subjects that we will present throughout the book, as we seek to present and understand people's experiences of living and dying with dementia and the service system that has developed to support them.

Numbers of people with dementia

Dementia is defined within Western health care as a syndrome, or collection of symptoms, that interferes with social and independent living (Ballard 2000). Epidemiological research estimates that worldwide 24 million people live with dementia and this number is forecast to be 81 million by 2040 (Ferri *et al.* 2005). There are differences in expected rates of increase, with numbers in developed countries forecast to rise by 100 per cent between 2001 and 2040, while those in India, China, South Asia and the western Pacific are forecast to rise by 300 per cent (Ferri *et al.* 2005). Central to the explanation of this increase is an overall increase in life expectancy, again more evident in some countries, but also a world trend. Figures from the UK underline this connection between increased age and numbers with dementia. The prevalence rate increases with age from 1 in a 1000 for 40–65 year olds to 1 in 5 for people over 80 years old (Alzheimer's Society 2006).

In the United States, it was estimated that, in 2000, 4.5 million people were living with Alzheimer's dementia. This figure represents a doubling of the recorded incidence since 1980 (Herbert *et al.* 2003) and it is predicted that by 2050 this figure will rise to between 11.3 and 16 million. Approximately 1.1 million of these people live with moderate to severe dementia and it is estimated that by 2015 this will rise to 2.8 million. In the UK, dementia affects 750 000 people (Alzheimer's Society 2006). Eighteen thousand people affected by dementia are less than 65 years old. The estimates are that by 2010 there will be 870 000 people with dementia. In Australia, population estimates published in 1998 identified 134 000 people with dementia. In the population aged 65–84 years, 5 per cent of people were affected, and for people over 85 years, this rose to 25 per cent (Australian Institute of Health and Welfare 1998). By 2002 overall numbers had risen to 162 000 (Giles *et al.* 2003). It is projected by 2040 there will be 500 000 people with dementia and by then dementia is expected to be the primary cause of major chronic illness in Australia.

The figures we have presented capture the irony of increased longevity. They are figures of particular relevance to the age cohort of most people reading this book (and of its authors). The current generation will live with this level of dementia as they grow old. Those of us who live into our 80s and 90s will find every fourth or fifth person will have dementia. Dementia is a subject that is crucial to us as citizens who have to decide on resource allocation. It is crucial to us as members of families who may have to make decisions about how to care for our parents, our siblings, and our partners. It is crucial to us as individuals as we contemplate meaning and identity in later life and as we consider the time we have to do the things we wish to do and the care we may need.

However, the figures may also reveal another significant level of meaning. Perhaps the simple juxtaposition of increasing longevity and numbers of people with dementia does not capture the whole picture. One reason is that certain presentations are now more likely to be named as being dementia. In the past similar characteristics may have been identified using a different term – senility, for example – or an explanation from a different epistemology may have been sought (Fox 1989, 2000), for example from an epistemology of mysticism or spirituality. Different terminologies to categorize the behaviours identified as dementia may be present in societies that are not suffused by Western epistemologies of science.

Moving from the epidemiological, it is also likely that the subjective perception of the meaning of the symptoms that together constitute dementia will vary over time and will change in relation to specific circumstances. It is not just long ago and far away that things are seen differently. People carry clusters of explanatory constructs that exist in a layered way in consciousness and it is these they bring to bear when asked to assess the meaning of social actions, or to ascribe an explanation to the manifestation of a particular symptom. These meanings and explanations jostle for prominence – for example, in times of stress there may be fissures created in what is believed rationally and other explanations for the challenges a person is confronted with will be sought. A person may profess a scientific rationalism when asked to explain their belief system but will invoke malign fate as being the cause of a trauma they are confronted with.

It is estimated that approximately 100 000 people with dementia die each year in the UK (Bayer 2006). However, life expectancy can be unpredictable. The time from an initial presentation of first symptoms of dementia[1] to death varies from about 2 to 20 years (Volicer et al. 1987), with fewer years expected

---

[1] There can be a considerable gap, often of some years, between first symptoms and a diagnosis. We will examine this and its potential impact on care planning and user involvement in Chapter three.

for those who develop dementia later in life (Brookmeyer *et al.* 2002). As the dementia progresses it is more possible to predict a person's death with some accuracy (Neale *et al.* 2001).

The cause of death for people with dementia is not easily determined. Death certificates rarely record deaths as being caused by dementia and autopsies are rare. This lack of clarity with regard to dying with, as well as from, dementia is one factor that has contributed to a lack of a focus in terms of service provision to meet people's needs at the end of life. We have already said that a further factor is that the individual's needs associated with dying are ignored because people with dementia are seen as 'already dead'. There are also no reliable figures on the number of people who have dementia and another terminal illness such as cancer (de Vries 2003). The most commonly recorded causes of death in people with dementia in the UK are pneumonia, a cardio-vascular event or pulmonary embolism (Keene *et al.* 2001). Hence, it is suggested that dementia is as much an underlying cause as a direct cause of death (Michel *et al.* 2002). There is also a high incidence of fractures, increasing the risk of premature death (Hermans *et al.* 1989).

Cox and Cook (2002) propose that people die with dementia in one of three ways. They can reach the end of their life with dementia, but die from another condition. Others with dementia reach the end of their life with a complex mix of dementia and other medical conditions which together lead to their death. Finally, some live until their dementia is very advanced and die with the complications that this brings, most notably aspiration pneumonia as a result of dysphagia (swallowing problems) (Jolley and Baxter 1997).

Introduction to our arguments

In this book we will examine the intersection of life-world narratives with professional discourses. We are using the word discourse to mean a system-atized structure of significance supported by, and supporting, social power and narrative as a subjective account emerging from the lived experience of each individual. These meanings will be elaborated on, and illustrated, in subsequent chapters.

The Sufi saying with which we began the book reminds us of the impor-tance of the *and* when combining one thing *and* another, even when they are closely related things. A theme throughout the book is this idea of the 'and'. We examine many areas where there are different perspectives addressing the same area of concern. We have already done this, above, when we looked at the figures for the increased numbers of people with dementia and considered these using an epidemiological approach. We then suggested that the increase might be explained by a shift in what we define as dementia, an approach that concentrates on the epistemological. If we look at the significance of not just the figures but of the syndrome they are seeking to capture we also have to consider how they are interpreted by people. This led us to consider systems of meaning in relation to dementia that draw on subjective understandings. The way we have examined dementia prevalence figures therefore provides an insight into the approach we will bring to bear on a number of areas where we want to emphasize the challenge inherent in addressing connections, in addressing the *and*. We are not, however, intent on reconciling differences in a neat way – there is something that is messy about our subject areas and about our engagement with them. We begin by introducing some 'ands' concerned with the book's focus and then consider a final 'and', discourse and narrative, that belongs with a consideration of the methods by which we make our arguments.

Living and dying

Our title, *Living and Dying with Dementia*, was chosen to underline that you can live until you die with dementia. It also captures a realization that to be living with dementia is to be dying with dementia, in that dementia heralds a biological process leading to death. To have dementia does not stop people living – nor does it strip their complexity from them. Thinking about living and dying with dementia has to involve a number of dimensions. Dementia affects individuals, their family, the health and social care system in which they are supported and it affects society more generally. Thinking about living and dying with dementia cannot, therefore, just focus on health issues for any one individual: a consideration of broader social understandings is required.

In discussing living and dying with dementia we do not wish to diminish the physical and emotional stress felt by some of those caring for a person with dementia and by the person themselves. In arguing for living until you die we are not seeking to render dementia as anything less than demanding. However, we will argue that the sequestration of the dying, and of people with dementia, into a separate domain stops connections being made between the potential for positive experiences and the loss and disablement that are widely felt to be synonymous with dying and with dementia. A paradox of living life is that loss is one of the things that can bring meaning to life. Some of the narratives we present will illuminate this.

If we accept that dementia is a life-limiting and terminal condition then we need to examine what death means in this context. Conventionally, we see dying as a process and death as an event, but in relation to many chronic and terminal illnesses, death can become a process.[2] That is, it takes place in different domains of our lives, it occurs physically, socially, psychologically and spiritually. These experiences may occur simultaneously or sequentially and, if the latter, they can occur over many years. However, this process of death in different domains is not an inevitable consequence of dementia. We will explore how particular approaches in care, specifically a focus on preserving the self, may result in the amelioration of social, psychological and spiritual death, in Chapters 3 and 4 respectively.

The presence of dementia in a person means that that person has a condition that will be with them as they die, regardless of the 'identified' cause of death. If a person's physical dying is ignored because the focus is on living, that person will die poorly. If physical dying is prioritized and the other dimensions of the person who is still living are not considered that person will die poorly. There is a particular dilemma for people with dementia in that waiting until we know that a person is imminently dying is too late for personal (and family) preparation, for seeking to achieve psychological, social and spiritual resolutions, things perceived to be the hallmarks of the best care for the dying (see Chapter 5).

People with dementia typically experience a gradual death. This poses challenges for them, their families and society. What should be done, when, by whom and where? Some of the tools designed to help people prepare for their own deaths and take control of this process, for example Advanced Care Plans, present particular issues in relation to people with dementia. Assumptions about autonomy in the personal management of this process by a cognitively capable person cannot be directly transferred to people with dementia. We will critique assumptions about autonomy in relation to all dying, arguing that dying as a complex and multifaceted process challenges ideas about the possibility, and desirability, of assuming autonomy to be the defining principle and end point of good care (see Chapter 4). Dementia requires society to be imaginative not just about the end point of what is to be achieved but also about the means by which this is approached. For example, other ways to undertake the resolution of important social, psychological

---

[2] Some people equate change in their lives with a sort of dying. The sportsman whose career is ended by injury might describe themselves as going through a process of 'dying' as one sort of person, as a person with a particular social and self-identity. They may 'start another life', subsequently pursuing a different career. David Peace's novel *The Damned United* (2006), about footballer and then football manager Brain Clough, offers a particularly vivid example of the trauma of such a change.

and spiritual agendas that work via non-verbal communication may need to be identified.

Care for people with dementia and care for people who are dying

We argue that both care for people with dementia and care for people who are dying can contribute, each to the other, to help improve care for people living and dying with dementia. Integrating approaches is not easy. Following the development of a palliative care approach a lot is known about care for people who are dying and there is extensive literature on care for people with dementia, but combining them requires new sorts of understanding. We want to sound a wake-up call in two directions, for those who care for people with dementia to pay attention to dying, and those who care for people who are dying to include people with dementia.

Palliative care focuses upon supporting people as they live until they die from life-limiting illnesses. Its origins were in the modern hospice movement, which initially sought to meet the needs of people dying with cancer. From the establishment of the first inpatient institutions in the 1960s a range of hospice and palliative care services have developed including inpatient, day and home care services. Recent expansion and diversification in the specialty has sought to address the needs of people dying with conditions other than cancer (Addington-Hall 1998). More recently, in the UK and Europe, the palliative care needs of people with dementia have begun to be considered (Dorenlot and Fremontier 2006; Hughes *et al.* 2005; Robinson *et al.* 2005a; Small *et al.* 2006). This reflects earlier developments in the US in this area (see Volicer 1986).

Care provision for people with dementia represents a diverse mix of discourses from clinical medicine to person-centred care. To varying degrees these discourses view dementia as a bio-psychosocial condition requiring multidisciplinary and multiprofessional input. It is the connections between these perspectives that need to be grasped if we are to provide services that best reflect the needs of people with dementia and their families. Many individual specialties have played a role in shaping dementia care and will continue so to do. They provide tools for examining the signs and symptoms of dementia and they offer ways of intervention that can greatly enhance the lived experience of the illness. However, while necessary, the contribution of any one understanding is not sufficient – dementia is more than something that can be captured in any one epistemology. Problems arise, however, if one epistemology is dominant, if it becomes a discourse that can define the parameters of what is considered possible or legitimate.

Life-world and system world

In our consideration of the relationship between living and dying, and care of the dying and dementia care, we will distinguish between system world and life-world concerns. Critical theorist Jurgen Habermas distinguishes between the system world and the life-world and warns of the encroachment of the former into the latter (Habermas 1975). The system world encompasses the institutions of society, including the state and the market. Within this system world the dynamic of modernity has seen the emergence of capitalism, typified by instrumental rationality[3] and systemized and secured through money and the nation state, including the welfare state. The welfare state, according to Habermas, is secured through bureaucratic-administrative power. But there is also a world of intersubjectivity, constituted socially, the life-world. This includes everyday life, usual consensus formation, desires, needs, and fantasies. Conflicts arise at the seam of the system and life-world. The imperatives of the market, or of the bureaucratic-administrative welfare state, can infiltrate life-world contexts in such a way that can assimilate the life-world to one or other of the system imperatives. The result is that, 'Public affairs have come to be regarded not as areas of discussion and choice but as technical problems to be solved by experts employing an instrumental reason' (Craib 1992: 239). Further, the development of the welfare state means that whole areas of personal relationships become subjected to legal requirements or they become managed via medical procedures and protocols and thus are abstracted from their contexts. Expert cultures, each holding partial frameworks, are together contributing to a fragmented consciousness (Craib 1992). 'The internal colonization of the life-world by the system results', so Habermas argues, 'in the cultural impoverishment and fragmentation of everyday consciousness' (Habermas 1987: 355, quoted in Rundell 1991: 138). This colonization is not total – the life-world contains

---

3 Instrumental reason is a way of looking at the world, or a way of conceiving of knowledge, that sees the things in the world, or the knowledge we can access, as instruments, as means to achieve our ends. It is an approach that sees a tree as a source of paper for a book like this, not a thing of beauty to be enjoyed for itself. Craib offers a summary description if I operate according to instrumental reason: 'I do not see my students as people engaged in learning but as people who, if I impress them sufficiently, might be useful in furthering my career. I do not see my ability to understand people as something to be placed at their service but as a means by which I can persuade them to do what I want to do.' Instrumental reason defines what serves modernity, capitalism or bureaucratic power, as rational. That is the rational is instrumental in furthering the dominant system world assumptions. What does not further these is irrational – for example, choosing not to work or not participating in civic society (Craib, 1992: 211).

a permanent communicative potential through which protests and social movements are formed.

If there is potential for different forms of communication despite the effects of instrumental reason, there are also different ways of knowing that coexist within modernity. First, there is the sort of scientific reason that many assume to be synonymous with truth. This is closely allied with the physical sciences and with medicine. This is the reason of hypothesis, of experiment, of validation. It is characteristically reductionist – breaking things down and looking at their parts, and it is harnessed instrumentally, that is it is used to 'do' things to objects or to people. Secondly, there are patterns of action and knowledge that develop and proceed according to principles of moral–practical rationality and are validated in terms of how far they are seen to be normatively right. For example, much of civic, political and social life relies on shared social norms and on agreed ethical practices. What is done is accepted as right and true through the actions undertaken and the relationships people are involved in and is not assessed against the criteria of scientific reason. That is, it becomes a lived, an enacted, truth. It is this understanding of reason that Habermas and other critical theorists saw as being overtaken by instrumental reason in modernity/capitalism. A third sort of reason occurs when people make aesthetic judgements. Such judgements have their own expressive rationality. They make sense to us subjectively. These judgements are validated by identifying their truthfulness for people. We will argue that one of the things a focus on narratives and on subjective experiences illuminates is that both living with illness and caring for someone draws on moral–practical rationality and also has an aesthetic dimension. These different dimensions are evident in, for example, understandings of what constitutes a good death,[4] something we will explore in Chapter 6.

The argument that Habermas has developed over many years is a complex one. It draws us into a philosophical tradition that looks back to Kant. We will return to this tradition, and to Kant, in Chapter 4 to help us explore different ways of thinking about the ethics of care. Overall, Habermas' position has two main implications for our project in this book. First, it offers us guidance on the way we can structure what we will present. We will focus on the life-world and the system world in different chapters and we will point to the encroachment of each on the other throughout. Secondly, we will argue that different forms of

---

[4] Toscani *et al.* (2003) reports that interviewees in their study of dying and bereavement were concerned with the scene of death. An aesthetics of dying, including its visual representation in the scene of death, determines the quality of the memory that the deceased leaves to the living (see Bertman 1991 on the aesthetics of death).

reason have to be considered and that one should not collapse the experience of dying and living with dementia under just one, and especially not under the narrow positivism of scientific reason. Rather, one should seek truth out of the activity of trying to reach consensus, via developing a language that is 'oriented to observing inter-subjectively valid norms and linked reciprocal expectations' (Habermas 1979: 118; see also his theory of communicative action, Habermas 1984, 1987). It is in the praxis[5] of seeking to understand through an exploration of different positions that the value of our approach is realized.

Self and society

Examining living and dying with dementia requires us to consider deep-seated understandings of what is feared and therefore shunned, or hidden away, in society and what is assumed about the nature of self. As we will see in Chapter 4, it is the diagnosis of dementia and not the process of dying that can trigger a person's social death, because dementia is assumed to signal the death of the self. The self is more than a cognitive being, but people often act as if the person who is cognitively impaired is less than fully human. People with cognitive impairments are at risk of being excluded from normal interpersonal affirmation and interaction, as well as from valued social roles. We recognize that there has been a major impetus to develop innovations in theory in relation to dementia care that address this exclusion and challenge an assumption that a loss of self comes with living with dementia. There are also many examples of innovative practice to draw on to illustrate our presentation in this book. These are testament to the imagination and tenacity of many people – lay and professional – who have sought to help people with dementia live as fully as they can until they die, despite prevailing societal and professional assumptions. If dementia and dying pose particular problems for society, and for professions within it, then imaginative solutions in these areas offer insights that can be used both for other groups with complex health and social care needs and to critique society's attitudes to the importance of cognition in relation to the self more generally.

In our consideration of people living and dying with dementia we are addressing two things that represent great fears in society, a loss of self and a loss of life. What often happens with such fears is that they are pushed away. The dominant system world is focused on seeking cures. If a cure is not feasible it prioritizes control over care. It values efficiency and rationality. It marginalizes those who are no longer productive, or are no longer active consumers. It marginalizes those who it sees as not rational.

---

5 Praxis is the sort of experience that comes out of our engaging with our world, out of our actions, including our work.

It is conceptually and emotionally difficult to see the losses associated with dementia as playing a positive part in people's lives. However, there is to be seen in the life-world of people with, and affected by, dementia, signs of meaning and learning, which are brought into clearer focus by the certainty of personal mortality. It requires the juxtaposition of the concepts and the realities of both living and dying to make this possible.

Narrative and discourse

We will argue in this book that there are two ways to approach understanding dementia that can contribute to enhancing living until you die. The first is to seek to understand the subjectivity of the person with dementia – this we will explore via privileging narratives of experience. The second is to examine professional discourses, present in the system world, and consider how they exist alongside each other, how they relate to broader system-wide assumptions and how they interact with the subjectivity of the person with dementia and their families.

The system world may see people with dementia through a professional lens that focuses on one aspect of a person, for example, symptoms. In such a world behavioural characteristics as well as psychological, emotional and spiritual realities are at risk of being treated as, at best, signs illuminating symptoms and, at worst, as phenomena unworthy of regard. Beyond the individual with dementia, a focus on symptoms may narrowly define those close to a person with dementia, including their family members, as simply 'carers'. Such a narrow definition diminishes the activity and the persons undertaking it. Illich discusses what he sees as the problems of intransitive verbs, specifically to cope and to care. Casting someone as a carer implies care is something to be done. Actions are diminished as they are cast in functional or instrumental language. A person looking after their mother or their wife is not just an instrumental carer (see Twigg 2000, 2004).[6]

---

[6] Illich, in 1995, presented a conference paper titled 'Against Coping' (published with a different title as Illich, 1995). He pointed out that the term 'coping' as in 'coping with sickness' was of very recent origin. In premodern times, 'Sickness, like pain, disability, tiredness, and fear was suffered, borne, shared, alleviated, dreaded or cured' (p. 11). By the late 1960s to cope began to appear, now used as an intransitive verb, as a way of existence. It was used without the additional word *with*, 'coping flourishes within this epistemic void' (p. 12). 'The Orphic "know thyself" now reads "check how your system is coping"' (p. 13). It is impossible to pursue the art of living, or the art of enjoyment, or the art of suffering in a way that preserves the ego – the ego is recast as a system that can be shaped and controlled by 'hazardous medicalization, socially disabling professionalism, and a debilitating ritualism' (Illich, 1995: 12).

What might be called symptoms can be understood in different ways, as can the meaning of 'carer'. For example, what has been called disruptive behaviour might be seen as a communicative device and not as a symptom of dementia. Carers or caring might be seen in holistic and not in instrumental and reductionist ways, as something anyone can do rather than something some people are. This would allow close family members to be engaged with as people who are more than the narrowly defined carers others may classify them as. Shifting views in such ways can allow established practices to be questioned and different ways of working devised.

We will seek to devise an understanding of dementia that starts from the premise that we need to understand what people with dementia think and feel and then move forward from that to consider what they want and need. Help should then be structured accordingly. We propose that other people, both lay and professional carers for example, need to 'be with' people with dementia, recognizing they are sentient beings with psychological and social realities, before they 'do for' them. If this is not done, at best, people with dementia are 'done to' and at worst harm is done. Society's difficulty in accepting subjectivity, and 'being with', as factors to shape practice and policy is rooted in modernity and its elevation of a specific understanding of reason and knowledge. (The distinction between being with and doing for draws on the work of Buber (1970) and Bauman (1993) and we will return to it in subsequent chapters where we will support Bauman's identification of a stage of 'being for' as something that should precede being with (see Small *et al.* 2006: 383–5).)

Privileging subjectivity means seeking to shape our understanding of what it is like to live with dementia, and the needs associated with dying by starting from the experience of people with dementia and people living with, and caring for, people with dementia. We will seek to access various narratives of such experience available to us. Howard Brody described a narrative as a bridging performance connecting the teller and the listener, or in this book, the teller – whose narrative we have accessed via various routes – us as writers and you as readers (Brody 1994). When applied to health concerns, narrative

> provides meaning, context, and perspective for the patient's predicament. It defines how, why, and in what way he or she is ill. The study of narrative offers a possibility of developing an understanding that cannot be arrived at by any other means.
>
> (Greenhalgh and Hurwitz 1999: 48)

Listening to narratives reminds us that while meaning and significance can be shared, each story is different. An approach that starts with a person's narrative can build bridges between various disciplines which may not share a common professional language. We see narratives as providing both case history and case study, that is, giving stories of individual experience (history) and providing a route to try out theory building (study). We will use narratives from people with dementia and their family members and we will include fiction and poetry.

The narrative form primarily used here is the oral/verbal, constrained as we are by the confines of a book. We have incorporated, though, a strand of visual narrative in the book, through the inclusion of photographs by Hapé Smeele (Smeele 2002). His longitudinal work, undertaken in a supported housing environment for people with dementia in The Netherlands and also in Bhutan, offers us another way to understand experiences of living and dying with dementia and the giving and receiving of care. Smeele is one of a number of photographers to document lives of people with dementia (see Greenblat 2004). We present his photographs here without written comment. They speak with an authentic language of their own, although we do say a little more about Hapé's intentions in his work below.

We need to sound a word of caution. In an approach that utilizes subjectivity, accessed via narratives, we are aware that we must be careful not to simply construct narrative as a new orthodoxy defining a prevailing truth. We want to use narratives in addition to professional discourses, not privileging one over the other. In so doing we have to recognize that both narratives and discourses are presented in a socio-economic and a cultural context and we have to bring the same level of critical concern to them as we do to other ways of seeing and explaining. One way we will do this is to return throughout the book to the potential of postmodernism – an approach that respects the existence of a plurality of perspectives – and to critical theory, specifically that of Habermas, which gives us a way of considering the interface of the individual life-world and the context, or system world.

Of course shifting one's view is not simple. As authors we come to this writing with our own life experiences, worldview, values and intellectual predispositions, as we will outline below. While we have attempted to be explicit about these we will inevitably get caught in the assumptions of prevailing discourses. For example, we have already been a little too easy in our use of 'person with dementia'. It is a convenient but reductionist term, as is, a too easy use of 'carer'. Saint Augustine in his *Confessions* (Book Ten) described the race of men as 'curious to know the lives of others, slothful to amend their own' (quoted in Plummer 2001: 232). No doubt we will end with things for which we still need to make amends.

There are some things we are sure of. We want to take seriously the insights of 'living and breathing, embodied and feeling human beings' (Plummer 2001: x).

Further, we agree with Denzin, whose position is succinctly summarized in Plummer, that researchers

> should take sides; should study experiences that are biographically meaningful for the researcher; should attend to pivotal turning point experiences; should uncover and display models of truth, accuracy and authenticity; should privilege languages of feelings and emotions over those of rationality and science; should examine multiple discourses and should write multivoiced polyphonic texts, which include the researchers' own experience.
>
> (Plummer 2001: 13, see also Denzin 1992, 1997)

Introduction to the authors

Following Plummer and Denzin, we will write explicitly about ourselves in the next paragraphs. We each bring different personal and professional/academic experiences and interest to this book.

Neil Small arrived at an involvement in this book through his previous research and scholarship. He writes:

> My interests have been in social policy and social theory. This led to an involvement in research in the early years of the HIV/AIDS epidemic in the UK. Ethnographic work with people with AIDS, in this period, led to an engagement with issues of stigma and loss, and with death. This work was followed by studies that increasingly became focused on two themes; first, studies that sought to access people's subjective experience of living with a chronic or terminal illness; second, looking at the way innovative services had originated and become established in this area, a specific focus became the modern hospice movement. Thinking about living and dying with dementia, in the way we do in this book, brings together a number of these academic interests.

Katherine Froggatt's involvement reflects both personal and professional experiences in the field. Her first personal encounter with dementia occurred with her grandmother's death seventeen years ago.

Memories of Lucy Gresford-Jones: 1911–1989

> Today (8 May 2004) is the anniversary of my granny's death. She died in 1989, 15 years ago, in a nursing home in Sevenoaks, Kent. I remember I was working as a staff nurse on night duty at Charing Cross Hospital when I received a phone call late Friday night from my mother to say she was dying. As soon as I finished work that next morning I travelled down to Sevenoaks, to join my mother, her two sisters and various cousins who had gathered together at the nursing home.
>
> I will always remember the weekend we waited for Granny to die. The stroke she had suffered previously had left her very disabled; she had severe contractures of her arm and leg on the affected side. A combination of deafness, dementia and the stroke also meant that she latterly did not communicate with words. She just looked on bemusedly.

That Saturday and Sunday as she lay in her bed, in her ground floor room, the sun shone outside. It was a glorious May weekend when the trees were just bursting forth their leaves, that vivid new green, of leaves emerging to face the world outside from furled covers. My memory is of sitting on the grass outside her room, talking, planning, whilst people took it in turns to sit inside the room with her, as she lay in the bed.

I have other memories from that weekend of sitting with aunts, uncles, siblings and cousins, at my aunt's house. Again in the garden, with the sun shining, cherry blossom still on the trees, on a bench, planning her funeral service, making decisions about what would be sung and said, and who would do what. It seemed a healthy time, and one I was privileged to be part of. I went back for my final night duty shift of that week on the Sunday evening. She died on the Monday.

Her funeral the following week was memorable for the flowers. She had loved gardens and gardening and flowers were important to her. She lay in her coffin in the church next door to my aunt's house overnight and was surrounded by flowers, bouquets, wreaths, and displays. When you walked into the church it looked like a wedding was taking place. A celebration and joyous occasion, although sad to see her go. At the end of the funeral people were encouraged to take away one of the bouquets with them. A sharing out of all that had been brought.

Katherine continues:

My memories recounted here focus on the point at which she was dying and present a positive picture that has meaning for me. I do not know if that is how other members of her family, my mother and aunts would see it. They were probably much more aware and impacted by the ongoing changes in her life prior to this point than I was. Over the last ten years my research has taken me into care homes for older people and I have engaged with people living in such settings, of whom, some have had dementia. More recently my parents-in-law (Alan and Gwen Kidd) were both diagnosed and died with dementia. Accounts of their experiences are present in this book, drawn from writing that my husband (Hugh Kidd) and his sister (Alison Kidd) have undertaken about their parent's situation towards the end of their lives. The challenges we describe in this book, of engagement between people living with and caring for dementia, of looking beyond symptoms to the subjective experiences of the person, have been present in all these encounters. I have been required to move beyond tidy ideas to learning to be present in these situations. Maybe, within these various experiences are the Denzin-like pivotal moments that initiated and energized the writing of this book for me.

Murna Downs, another of the authors of the book, is both a daughter of someone who lived and died with dementia, and a Professor of Dementia Studies. She has had a long standing interest in the person's experience of living with dementia and in approaches to ensuring quality of life and quality of care for people with dementia and their families, focusing on primary care and long term care. In Murna's words:

I expect I was invited to write this book because of my position as Professor in Dementia Studies while my own motive and interest in writing the book was to learn about palliative care in order to be of most help to my mother, who died within a year of us starting the book. In writing this book I have drawn on my and family's experience of my mother's living and dying with dementia. In so doing I have been keen to find a philosophical, theoretical and empirical basis for how the changes she and we experienced served to enrich us all. She inspired us to look beyond the rational, honour the past, celebrate closeness, relish the moment, and trust in the meaning and order of life. I hope this book provides a vehicle to disseminate some of what she taught us to others.

Hapé Smeele, whose photographs are on the cover and at various points in the book, is a Dutch portrait and documentary photographer. Ten years ago he started on three pieces of work about 'the quality of life'. He started this from the point of view that people often talk too easily about others and their quality of life. It is seldom seen that people really pay attention to how these people themselves experience their lives. In 1997 his book *Een andere werkelijkheid* (*A different reality*) was published, a book about individuals with multiple learning disabilities. In 2002 the sequel to this book, *Met de moed van een ontdekkingsreiziger* (*With the courage of an explorer*) was also published. The subject of this book is dementia and dying. Both books were awarded several prizes. He is currently working on a book about Buddhists in the Netherlands and the way they give their source of inspiration a place in their daily lives. Hapé Smeele lives and works in Hilversum, The Netherlands.

Outline of the book

In Chapter 2, The life-world: journeys with dementia, we present the life-world of people with, and affected by, dementia primarily through narratives. We use the metaphor of a journey to structure this chapter. We recognize that the journey is an image used by policy-makers and professionals to describe the experience of people with a range of conditions, and there is a danger that it has been over-used. However, the metaphor is present in both people with dementia and family members' accounts of their experience and it provides a useful way to engage with these experiences from their perspective. Three elements of this journey are described: starting the journey, being on the journey and the journey's ending. The journey is a long one, often taking many years and incorporating many aspects of a person's life. Many incremental losses are described that shape a person's everyday experiences. Key points of transition are identified on this journey, where a person's life-world intersects with the system world of service provision. Of particular significance at this point is how the person is perceived in terms of 'self' (explored further in Chapter 4). We observe that there are paradoxical experiences in this interaction with services that mean that the person with dementia, and their family members, either receive too little or too much intervention from the system world.

In Chapter 3, The system world: developments in service provision, we present the way in which the system world attempts to meet people's needs when living and dying with dementia. Different professional discourses frame the focus of care for people with dementia and their families. In response to the perceived inevitability of the physical and cognitive decline that accompanies dementia a number of models of service provision have been developed. These are explored through an account of care for people with dementia including that provided by clinical medicine and person-centred care. We also examine care for people who are dying and identify implications for service provision. This book does not provide specific clinical advice on how to provide care for people who are dying with dementia. Several texts have recently been written that address the practicalities of clinical needs (Hughes 2006; Burns and Winblad 2006). Nor do we consider patterns of dementia and its care across the world. Most of our examples and the literatures we draw upon come from Western societies.

We argue that care for people with dementia has not fully engaged either with dying or with the losses a person with dementia and their family experience. Their focus has been on managing what are identified as symptoms in the person with dementia and dysfunctions in that individual's interactions with others. Historically, developments in care for people who are dying, including palliative care, have not engaged with the needs of people with dementia. However there is some evidence of this being addressed in specific services. We make the case that there is potential for integration of clinical medicine, person-centred care and palliative care and argue that if this were achieved it would overcome some of the limitations currently identified. One such limitation is that when dying is a consideration in service provision most services are focused on support for people with what is termed severe, advanced and end-stage dementia. This leaves much of what is provided for people with dementia not acknowledging the terminal nature of the condition, even from its earliest stages.

Chapter 4, Self and autonomy, explores ways in which we understand the self and the reasoning that leads us to assume a loss of self in dementia. Where self is seen to be lessened by cognitive changes resulting from dementia there are implications for the person in terms of how they are involved in managing their own life and in what is provided with, and for, them. We will explore the implications of reinstating subjectivity and we will support an argument that the self is retained even when a person lives with dementia. We offer ways of critiquing the importance of autonomy of self.

We then move in Chapter 5, Quality of care and quality of life, to consider how the way services are currently focused reflects values associated with particular perceptions of quality. These perceptions reflect a number of viewpoints that might not take into account the experiences of the recipients of services. In this way this builds on the argument in Chapter 4. Assumptions inherent in the way quality is perceived emphasize individualism, autonomy and utilitarianism. There is also an assumption made about a linear relationship between quality of care and quality of life that can be questioned. We offer an alternative way to understand quality of life and care from the person with dementia's perspective. Building on existing work, we offer an approach that locates quality in the relationships we have with those around us, and in the society in which we live, as an alternative to an efficiency-based and individualistic way of assessing services.

A broader perspective on dying in society is the focus of Chapter 6, The 'good death' and dementia. Here we provide a further explanation for the experiences of people living and dying with dementia. Each person's experience is shaped by the coming together of different social discourses: ageing, disease and dying. As these are currently constituted each have negative consequences for people with dementia.

The process of ageing has different meanings, ranging from a normal process, a process to be managed and a process to be fought against. Common to many of the understandings of ageing is a lack of recognition of dying as its inevitable end point. An interest in intervention and cure, characteristic of mainstream medicine, seeks to manage diseases. The person with dementia or the person deemed to be dying who cannot be cured is left isolated. Death is seen as a failure. This denial of dying and the sense that death is feared and has to be controlled shapes the presence of a 'good death' template in any society. The importance of this good death template is discussed with reference to different models that have been prominent in specific historical periods. What is a good death changes to reflect shifting societal values, and could change again.

In Chapter 7, Looking forward, we draw the arguments of previous chapters together. Living and dying with dementia requires a broad perspective in terms of both when help is needed and what focus that help should have. Attention to dying needs to be integrated into an engagement with people with dementia and their families from their early encounters with the social and health care system. However, this also needs to be mirrored in the broader policy world and in society more generally. We present principles that could be used to plan and deliver services that start with the individual with dementia and their family but look out to all people around the person with dementia. In order to provide a 'good' death for people with dementia, we need to create a good dying which is worked out individually, within services, and collectively, within society.

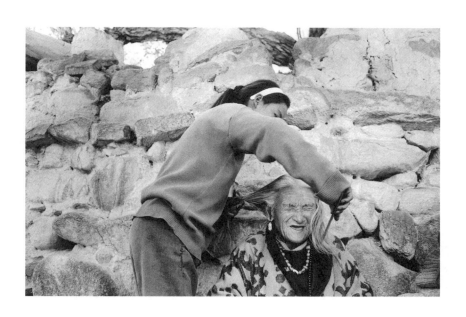

Chapter 2

The life-world:
Journeys with dementia

We are travelling from an old life to a new.
Pat, James and Ian (downloaded from
http://www.alzscot.org/downloads/dontmake.pdf)

Introduction

In our first chapter we identified system world and life-world concerns that would structure the way we approach our examination of living and dying with dementia. In this chapter, our focus is on the life-world, specifically on the journey taken by the person with dementia and by their families, friends and carers. This life-world experience of living with dementia is complex. It is embedded in the wider system world of organizational structures, as we begin to identify. Our challenge in this chapter is to present life-worlds in a way that captures the individuality and heterogeneity of people's experience, but also recognizes that many aspects of the life-world will display common features for people with dementia and their family members.

We have chosen to draw on the metaphor of 'journeys' to describe different features of the dementia experience, from living to dying. We have chosen this metaphor because it is commonly used in palliative care and is also present in the dementia care world. It is also used by people with dementia (Davis 1989; Noyes 2004), by their family members (McGowin 1994; Caracciolo 2006), and self-help organizations (see http://www.vch.ca/dementia; http://www.alzscot.org). We describe three phases: starting the journey, being on the journey and the journey's ending. These phases are not distinct, there are many overlaps. We present them as distinct here only as a heuristic device to help us structure our argument.[1]

---

[1] It is an issue resonant of controversy both in dementia care and bereavement care as to whether the identification of stages (or phases) is a useful conceptual device. Often it is the rhetorical convention that imposes structure that can be misused to produce a crude guide to practice whereby people are encouraged to go through prearranged (and for them arbitrary) stages. See Kúbler-Ross's (1969) stages of dying. We will return to this issue in Chapter 3.

If there are three phases there are, in our considerations, also three dimensions of journeys with dementia that exist within each stage. First, as far as we can from the person with dementia's perspective, we describe what it is like to live with dementia. This includes a consideration of the inner psychological, emotional and spiritual journeys that occur for people in response to the changes they experience. Secondly, we move outward, beyond the person with dementia to those people around them and their experiences of being alongside the person with dementia. Thirdly, we consider the physical and social environment, the spaces and places people with dementia and their family encounter during their journeys. This final dimension also makes reference to how this social context shapes people's experiences.

The journey with dementia is characteristically a long one which encompasses many cognitive and functional changes that are associated with progressive nature of the dementias. There are significant points of interaction between life-worlds and the system world, in the main, through the support services received. These interactions can fundamentally shape people's experiences, sometimes positively, often negatively. Common issues include concerns about the everyday impact of dementia on a person's opportunities, interactions and on their identity, the nature of services and how they are structured, and the way we manage dementia and the boundary between life and death in society.

Journeys for the person with dementia

The journey with dementia often begins with small changes noticed by a person, or by people close to them. It may be many months, or even years, before the changes are named as being linked to dementia. Subsequently, characteristic of the journey are a series of changes, often framed as losses. They make themselves visible in everyday living both for a person with dementia and for those around them. The varied functional, cognitive, psychological, emotional and social consequences of dementia for an individual may lead to a need for support and assistance either in a person's home, or via a move to a more supported setting. The final phase, where an individual is dying, can occur at any point on this journey, not just when the dementia condition is deemed to be of an advanced nature.

An academic and professional interest in the day-to-day experience of people with dementia is a relatively recent phenomenon. It has only been since the early 1990s that a concern with understanding this experience has been present in mainstream literature (e.g. Cotrell and Schulz 1993: Downs 1997). Since then a considerable body of literature on what it is like to live with dementia has developed (see Clare 2003; Friedell 2003; Keady and Keady 2005; Killick and Allan 2001; Harris 2002; Phinney 2002; Pratt and Wilkinson 2003; Sabat 2001). Most of this literature focuses on the early stages of dementia, drawing on people with dementia who are both verbally articulate and coherent (Downs 1997). Moving beyond the early experiences of living with dementia there are descriptions of progression, in particular for younger people (Boden 1998; Keady and Nolan 1994). In interviews with ten younger people with dementia Keady and Nolan identified nine stages of experience: slipping, suspecting, covering up, revealing, confirmation, maximizing, disorganization, decline and death. We will comment on these stages as they relate to different parts of the journey with dementia.

Starting the journey

There is a growing evidence base to suggest that people are aware of the difficulties they are experiencing before the condition is diagnosed (Froggatt 1988; Moniz-Cook *et al.* 2006): because of their awareness of their experiencing memory loss, Keady and Nolan (1994) describe this as slipping. Eliciting the meaning of dementia for people who suspect they may have the condition, prior to diagnosis, reveals that they see a sense of a potential for the loss of self, a loss of control over bodily functions which they associate with an anticipated sense of shame, the foreseen inevitability of long-term care, and decline associated with a loss of pleasure (Moniz-Cook *et al.* 2006). People beginning to experience cognitive symptoms and functional impairments describe a concern with 'losing their mind' or 'going mad', as is described in this account by a person with dementia:

> Looking back, I think I probably knew that something was wrong. The signs were there ... the memory lapses, the confusion, the angry outbursts. I guess there's knowing, and then there's knowing.
>
> Vancouver Coastal Health Dementia Stories, downloaded from
> http://www.vch.ca/dementia/problems_story.htm, 25 November 2006

For younger people with dementia, the place of work is likely to be a significant area where the dementia experience is lived out and where it may be most obviously present initially. People's responses to the realization that something is wrong may lead to the adoption of practical strategies to manage their lives, so that others do not notice the changes. This is a process that has been termed 'covering up' by Keady and Nolan (1994), and may include a withdrawal from situations where social interaction is too overwhelming, perhaps because of its speed or nature.[2] The use of lists and notes to manage memory problems are adopted by some people.

---

[2] In the UK the surprise resignation of Prime Minister Harold Wilson in 1976 (then aged 60) is now generally understood as resulting from his realization that the memory losses he was experiencing were indications of the early stages of Alzheimer's disease. He died of colon cancer in 1995.

An accumulation of various small changes in an individual's abilities can lead to the person themselves, or family members, beginning to discuss what is happening. This is the stage Keady and Nolan (1994) call 'revealing'. It is a stage that can lead to an engagement with health care professionals (usually doctors and nurses) to establish a cause for what is experienced or observed. These early encounters with the system world, often ongoing over a period of time, can lead to formal assessments to determine and confirm a diagnosis of dementia (Keady and Nolan 1994). This experience of being assessed for dementia has been described, by Keady and Gilliard (2002), as being for many a negative one, being threatening to one's sense of self and one's coping. Bernard MacLaverty's short story *The Assessment*, set in an assessment ward of a hospital, provides us with insight into how it might feel to be under scrutiny, believing people are watching for the mistakes you make [3]

> They're watching me. I'm not sure how – but they're watching me. Making a note of any mistakes. Even first thing in the morning, sitting on the bed half dressed, one leg out of my tights. Or buttoning things up badly. Right button, wrong buttonhole. Or putting the wrong shoe on the wrong feet. I don't think there's a camera or anything, but I just can't be sure'.
>
> (MacLaverty 2005: 61)

A diagnosis formalizes what has been experienced and provides a way to explain and make sense of these experiences. However, a diagnosis also names the experiences in relation to the medical system world. As we describe in Chapter 3, dementia can be understood in different ways dependent upon the profession one encounters. The way it is viewed has consequences for the person with dementia, not least in terms of their experiences of care.

Being on the journey

Being on the journey involves moving on, from the point at which dementia is recognized as being present, through more diverse terrain as the progressive loss of abilities are encountered. Each change requires adjustment, accommodation and assimilation. While these changes may lead to emotional reactions such as fear, people can also find meaning and richness in them. As noted by Keady and Nolan (1994), this period may be characterized by 'maximization', learning to live with the different changes that ensue.

---

[3] In the UK the onset of dementia and then its consequences began to feature prominently in popular culture in the early years of this century. Specifically, it has shaped key story lines in radio and TV's longest running soap operas, respectively *The Archers* and *Coronation Street*.

Rich descriptions of living with dementia are provided by Phinney and Chesla (2003) and others (see Bryden 2005). Phinney and Chesla interviewed and observed nine people with mild to moderate dementia and their family caregivers over a period of two to six months. People were asked to describe what it was like to live with Alzheimer's dementia. From these accounts and their own observations, the researchers identified the way in which dementia is experienced in, and through, the lived body. They propose three ways in which the bodily experience of living with dementia is manifested: 'being slow', 'being a blank' and 'being lost'. These sorts of experiences are seen in other accounts too.

'Being slow' is about the way in which a person's body slows down. Activities and conversations that would formerly have never been thought about, but just happened, become much more laborious and stilted. Bryden (2005), who has lived with dementia for over ten years, describes an ongoing tiredness and struggle to continue to hold onto her life. She uses the image of a swan serenely gliding through the water which represents her presentation of self to the world, whilst underneath the swan's legs are frantically paddling just to keep going. The frantic movement, like whatever is happening in her brain, may not be visible to anyone. The image of treading water is also used to capture the effort that can be expended, when living with the changes dementia brings, in trying to stay where one is.

Phinney and Chesla's respondents report the experience of *'being a blank'*. This is manifested, both in mind and body, through forgetfulness of memories and what is described as 'bodily silence'. With forgetfulness people cannot remember specific information or are unable to reflect on events and memories of events. Metaphors of searching for what has gone are invoked: 'Ivy says, "Well, if I've lost me memory I must go and dig, dig some fo foal, coal out somewhere, see if I can get some, gotta get me coal cart" ' (Ivy Redburn, in Bruce *et al.* 2002: 73). Other metaphors used are of being in a blizzard or a fog. For example, Bryden describes herself as feeling 'foggy in my head' (Bryden 2005: 97).

Whilst people with dementia may have difficulty with recall they may still retain their ability for recognition and have implicit memory for events, that is, memories which are not accessible to conscious awareness, but which nevertheless affect their behaviour or their response to a person or event (Sabat 2006a). For example, Baldwin (2006a) describes the example of a lady who frequently took away the tea trolley where she lived. Her previous experience of being in charge of a voluntary team that provided refreshments at a local hospital was an implicit memory. This memory was an impetus to engage meaningfully with the tea trolley, that is take it around the home, providing drinks for people living there.

Bodily silence and stillness may be experienced by a person with dementia and reflects the difficulties with activities just described. We see this 'being a blank' in a blog account, '*So I'm Demented*', written by a 50-year-old American woman recently diagnosed with dementia. She describes the impact dementia has in various ways in her life.

> In my moments of clarity, all seems fine and well. Then there is the rest of the time … wandering around the house trying to figure out what I'm supposed to be doing, asking my poor husband for the umpteenth time 'this is Monday, right?' ('no, dear, it's Tuesday and that's the seventh time you've asked since lunch'), checking and rechecking my list of what I'm supposed to do today – then not doing it because I forget again, finding taps running and things put in odd places, *sitting and staring then wondering what I was just thinking about* … welcome to my nightmare …
>
> Posted by ummzibba (http://buzzfrommybrain.blogspot.com/) (our emphasis)

'*Being lost*' manifests itself for people with dementia in three ways: being lost in the spatial world, being lost with equipment and being lost in activities. People with dementia may find themselves less sure about the physical environment. This can affect their ability to negotiate travelling from one place to another, even on routes that have been travelled frequently, for example, the walk to local shops. There may even be difficulties in smaller spaces such as rooms, for example being sure how to exit them:

> On another occasion when my Mum and Dad came to visit me in a cottage I was renting in Scotland, I remember my Mum asking me how she could get out of the room and saying, 'There are far too many doors here'.
>
> Murna Downs

Journeys of all scales can be affected. A person with dementia about continuing to live at home on his own captures some of this: 'Every morning when I wake up, I'm unsure where I am and feel anxious. But when I see familiar things, I know I'm at home', John, as told to Denise Williams (Alzheimer's Society 2003: 18).

People with dementia were also observed by Phinney and Chesla (2003) as being unable to recognize the world of objects, that is, objects that were a part of daily life, for example, spectacles or handbags. Despite being in their normal place, they were just not 'seen' or 'recognized' for what they were. As we saw in Umzibba's blog, forgetfulness in terms of things, events and objects is a reflection of this experience of being lost. People may also be lost in the world of activity and find it difficult to remember procedures necessary to do tasks that were previously easily undertaken.

'Being lost' can result in people finding ways to manage the uncertainty this experience creates. This can be seen in the routines people with dementia establish to enable them to live their daily life and to manage their spaces and activities, as John recounts here:

> My independence is hugely important to me. I might seem a prisoner to my routines. I can't just pop out, I can't do my job or go for a drive, but I still manage to live on my own, manage my affairs and exercise my freedom of choice. It can be a struggle but, even if this don't always go right, it's worth it.
>
> John, as told to Denise Williams (Alzheimer's Society 2003: 19)

A further aspect of being lost is the extent to which people with dementia experience a loss of who they are. The image of being lost, present in metaphors used by people with dementia to talk about their experiences, can refer to someone having lost something tangible, as Ivy talked about earlier. The loss of a person's mind is described as 'slipping away'. The concern with how the self may change is implicitly described by Boden (1998) in the title of her book 'Who Will I Be When I Die?'.

People's experiences of day-to-day life are also inextricably bound up with their social context. Relating and communicating, within that context, is an integral aspect of how life is experienced (MacQuarrie 2005). Holst and Hallberg (2003) describe how people with dementia talk about their difficulties in continuing to relate to other people, because of problems of not being able to remember their names and the awkwardness that ensues when they have to keep asking the person. Relationships can be intimate contacts, one-to-one interactions with other people in their social network and also fleeting encounters with the wider community that they live within. Lyman (1998) identifies how people with dementia's awareness of how others react to them can be the most difficult part of living with cognitive changes. Here John describes how he is able to negotiate with, and be supported by, local networks in his community: 'I keep to places and shops I know well. Some shop staff know about me and I trust them to help. I've got a mobile phone and can call a friend if I get in trouble', John, as told to Denise Williams (Alzheimer's Society 2003: 18).

Both formal organizations (the system world) and informal local groups (the life-world) are not always prepared, or able, to make space for people with dementia. There is a process of social exclusion that can be observed. For example, whilst some faith groups do address care for people with dementia, local churches, synagogues, mosques and other religious places of worship are not always equipped to provide a space for them (Goldsmith 2004). As Ummzibba describes, her fellow believers are not able to adjust to the changes in her.

> Really, what is there to say when one cannot grasp the essence of what is being discussed? I am really dreading Friday. Supposed to meet with the Muslim sisters.

They want to start helping each other memorize parts of the Qur'an. I know this will be impossible for me. I also know they will not understand ... if only they will just let me come and enjoy their company. No one can understand this unless it is happening to them. A mind is really a terrible thing to lose.

Posted by ummzibba (http://buzzfrommybrain.blogspot.com/)

For people with dementia, the ability to be proactive in the maintenance of social links may no longer be possible (Holst and Hallberg 2003). They require others to be with them in their social network and to support them in a new way.

Alison Kidd's account of taking her parents sailing illustrates how revisiting former activities can impact on a person's sense of self. It demonstrates that sense of self can be affirmed by a familiar social context and interaction, where each person knows their place.

My brother and I attempted to take both our parents down to Salcombe where they had always had their much-loved sailing holidays. We managed a short sail with the two of them on my 20 foot boat and that went really well – my father, at the helm, looked as if he'd already arrived in heaven – he had a huge smile which stretched from ear to ear as he revelled in being back in a boat and sailing again. It was worth all the miles of driving and hassle just to see that. My mother (surprisingly) seemed really happy – wedged in by one or both of us when the boat heeled (inevitable as my father relished the strengthening breeze!) – when we tacked, she happily reached out to help with the jib sheets – the old familiar actions of years of being a crew being hardwired in her brain. ... Maybe she was happy because the context was so familiar and her role within it – or maybe she was just happy because she sensed how happy my father was and she knew, at some level, that her condition created so many tensions for him.

Alison Kidd

This sailing trip provided a social context where roles and self were restored to how they had been in many previous experiences. Familiar activities and responses were resumed with the consequences of cognitive and functional impairment on daily living receding into the background.

As a person with dementia has increased problems in comprehending what is happening to them, communication and engagement is more challenging for all concerned. While there are neurological reasons for a person's communication difficulties (for example their difficulty in finding the correct word) much has been written about how interactions with people with dementia also inhibit their capacity for communication (Cheston and Bender 1999; Killick and Allan 2001; Kitwood 1997a). Hugh Kidd recounts how he managed to find ways to engage with his mother, Gwen, in her distress.

One day, in the early stages of my mother's dementia when she was almost constantly confused and distressed, she couldn't be left. Alison and I had come home to help because Alan was leading a service. The trouble was that Alan was confused and unprepared for the service. Today I felt unable to face the embarrassment of sitting in the congregation with long and painful silences and much paper shuffling. Alison agreed to take this one on. This left me with the task of being with Gwen and preparing lunch for us all.

I found this relatively short stage of her decline when she was almost continually distressed very difficult. She was tearful and calling out and restless. I couldn't bear seeing her like this. Having the practical task of preparing lunch was a relief. Finding ways to ease her pain was more difficult. She wandered unhappily.

There was a short period of relative ease with some communication then. For some reason she sat down in the lounge. I went on trying to prepare the meal but at the same time made frequent visits into the lounge. Every time I put my head round the door and waved to her – she waved back. Communication – sometimes almost a smile through the distress! Every couple of minutes, I put my head round the lounge door and, in between these visits, called out cheerfully to her from the kitchen. For a while there was connection and some relief from her distress for us both.

Hugh Kidd

This account illustrates some of the emotional distress experienced by and for a person with dementia, as seen by her son. What is described here is a need for reassurance and affirmation that everything is all right, in both verbal and non-verbal ways. Later on in Gwen's life, when she was no longer living at home but had moved into a care home, her daughter, Alison Kidd, writes about several occasions when non-verbal communication did or did not occur.

At a rehabilitation nursing home, the first time (in my life) that M (Gwen) stared blankly through me. Painful. How could I get her to look at me again?

After I had taken M to the residential care home for the first time from Norfolk – we had something to eat and then the care staff transferred M to her bed to rest and left me to say 'goodbye' to her – I went in and M looked wide-eyed and terrified and she clutched my hand and held onto it really tightly in a 'please don't leave me here in this strange place where I don't know where I am' way. She wouldn't let go. I found that really difficult.

Arriving at the residential care home in the middle of their morning service and quietly creeping in the back – (D (Alan) nodding off and dribbling in his chair) M (bright-eyed) spotting me immediately and just staring at me throughout the rest of the service – not smiling but staring in a lovely 'I know you – you're my daughter' way that was really heart warming – her stare (across the room) was so intense that others were noticing it and smiling.

I think it was her birthday and there was cream cake – M was sticking both hands in it and kneading it as well as eating it – cake was going everywhere, but it didn't matter and there was a celebratory spirit to it.

Wheeling M in her wheelchair into the town to walk around the shops – M showed no interest or engagement even when I stopped the chair and picked up flowers for her to smell or pointed out birds. I was disappointed. When we got back, I parked the wheelchair next to a seat in the care home garden (it was very sunny) and stretched out on the seat to doze in the sun for a bit and think about things. I suddenly felt someone straighten the collar of my shirt and pat it down in place – it was M but in the moment of me opening my eyes, she was already withdrawn again. But I felt we had communicated.

M 'stealing' the food off a fellow resident's plate at the residential care home. They had to move her in the end because she kept doing this. I felt rather proud of her!

When M wasn't well or resting on her bed I, several times, climbed up beside her and just lay quietly next to her – either snoozing myself or just being and hoping she would enjoy the familiarity of someone next to her in bed.

Taking her freesias in the hopes that she would enjoy smelling them and putting them in a vase only for her to stare blankly into space.

Alison Kidd

These cameos of communication and relating illustrate the mixture of ways in which family members interact and the losses, endings and meanings found that are experienced in many small ways, as well as in the larger more obvious ones. There is a growing body of research evidence suggesting that people with significant cognitive and functional loss continue to be capable of communication and connection with others (Norberg 1998, 2001; Killick and Allan 2001). In situations like this communication and the way in which a relationship is sustained can be based on subtle interactions. We will return to this in Chapter 3.

Ending the journey

Muriel braves the blizzard with her big blue eyes.
In a few more weeks, though, Muriel Prior dies.
For the men and women written on this board
Death's got the only door-code out of Whernside ward
And till Rene Parker died, Rene died,
her husband's weekly kisses consoled his bride.
Only eight more kisses then he'll lose his dear,
swept off in the blizzard where brides disappear.
Eight more weeks for Matthew Paul, who says GO AWAY
to the blizzard worsening every day.
Though the blizzard's blowing, right until the last
he'll sing 'Daisy, Daisy' through the stormy blast.

From *Black Daisies for the Bride* (Harrison 1993: 26–7) (sung to the tune of 'In the Bleak Midwinter')

'*Black Daisies for the Bride*', from which this song comes, is a play written about life in a former long-term hospital facility for people with dementia in the north of England. The song captures the inevitable outcome that people with dementia will encounter – their death. This physical, bodily, death of the person, an event that commonly occurs after many years of living with the dementia, whilst a tangible event, is not the only way in which dying can be understood. As we argue later, in Chapter 6, for people with dementia the boundary between life and death is diffuse and entails more than their physical death.

A person with dementia may die socially as well as physically (Cox and Cook 2002), and the presence of dementia can be more or less significant in shaping people's experiences of dying and death, dependent upon its progression and the other medical conditions present. For a person with dementia who dies shortly after being diagnosed while the illness is in its early stages, their dying will be more shaped by other underlying causes rather than the dementia. Other people die with multiple medical conditions where dementia plays a more significant part in shaping their experiences. A person may also die with the consequences of dementia dominating their experience. Often, dying is long and slow and preceded by a recognizable period of decline (Keady and Nolan 1994) where formal care is required. It is not always easy to determine when a person is dying. The process of deterioration, although inevitable, can occur over a period of months and years, until finally a person dies. The period at the end-of-life just before a person dies is often characterized by the person being confined to their chair or bed and becoming withdrawn, unable to communicate verbally and dependent on others for all their personal care and eating and drinking needs. Federica Caracciolo (2006) describes this phase in her husband's life:

> One Sunday, not having found him in the communal lounge where the patients gathered for recreation in the afternoons, I went up to his room. He was sitting in an armchair, one arm connected to a drip and tied to the arm of the chair to keep it from falling. His breathing had become very laboured. Although his temperature had gone down, he was in a state of extreme weakness. The doctor told me that he had not eaten for two days and they wanted to begin force-feeding. I strongly opposed this, deeming that Francesco had suffered enough.
>
> (Caracciolo 2006: 106)

This physical death of a person with dementia is an important part of the experience of the journey for family members. The nature of the death may colour how the whole journey is then regarded in retrospect. The notion of peace being achieved for the person who has died is important to many people, and family members sometimes describe the death as being a relief for the person with dementia. Alan Bennett describes his mother's death as being one that reflected how she lived.

> In the event her death is as tranquil and unremarked as one of those shallow ripples licking over the sands that I had watched so many times from her window. All her life she has hoped to pass unnoticed and now she does
>
> (Bennett 2005: 120)

In describing her experiences of her parents' journeys with dementia, Alison Kidd here recounts taking her father Alan to visit his wife, Gwen. They now lived in separate care homes and this visit was arranged as Gwen was very frail and thought to be dying. Alison thought this would be the last time Alan would see her. After some time together as a family, they left Alan with Gwen and then came back to say good-bye.

> After a while, we went back in and gently suggested to our father that we would have to leave soon. When my brother and I were prompting him about saying 'goodbye' – aware that this really might be the long goodbye, Alan said to her '*I don't need to say "goodbye" to you Gwen because I will be with you for ever and ever and ever*'. I think we realized at that moment that he did grasp the finality of the situation and yet, it was lovely, that his previous anger, grief and confusion about losing her (or being separated from her) had all gone – he seemed happy and at peace with her in a way we hadn't seen for a year maybe. I think he could cope with her dying better than he could cope with her being separated from him in life by her dementia.
>
> Alison Kidd

As the above account illustrates, in relationships where both people live with dementia, knowing and communicating the knowing about dying does occur. In the complicated situations that exist in families where dementia is present for more than one person, relationships and communication becomes strained and pressured in ways not necessarily imagined earlier in life. Additional experiences for family and friends, bereaved because of the physical death of a person, are described later.

The inner journeys

The bad home

> God so loved the world
> but he did not love this place.
> All I want to do is die.
> So why can't I be let to do so?
> Why can't you just lay down your head?
>
> I walk and walk and walk
> but there is no God,
> not in this place.
> This is The Bad Home –
> He has forgotten its existence.
>
> I get up and walk till I fall.
> Sinful though I be
> I'll ask God for His mercy.
> I'm too old to do anything.
> I'm just a dustbin.

It's all the same here.
Some of the girls grasp you
as if you're a cat or a dog.
They're too young. They can't
understand the problems of age.

It's all the same here.
They're so busy,
they'll help you into anything,
even rags. You're not a person
when you come in here.

Nothing to do, nothing to say.
It's all blackness in front of me.
Another thing, they just sit there
and turn their thoughts inward.
That's why we'll never get better.

God so loved the world
But He doesn't love me.
I used to be happy,
but now I'm angry with Him
because I'm still here.

(Killick and Cordonnier 2000)

People with dementia are seen by some writers as being engaged in an inward journey of sense-making about what is happening to them (Lyman 1998; Sabat 2001). Here we consider two strands to this inward journey: people's awareness of what is happening to them in the present and their awareness of what this means for their future. The poem by Killick and Cordonnier engages with both strands, although the strands are not always easily distinguishable. Elizabeth Cohen describes the way in which dementia and death are intertwined in her father's visit to a doctor.

> Dr Eder says that it would be good to keep Daddy busy. Daddy needs clocks and calendars, signs and symbols, points of reference. I should write pertinent information on sheets of paper for him.
> I tell Dr Eder about the memory project. How we go over one set of memories each night. 'Could that help him, that sort of thing?' I ask.
> 'I don't know, couldn't hurt. Just be aware it's a progressive illness. It might not be today or tomorrow or this week, but he will go downhill. He will get worse. And you need to start thinking about what you are going to do then.'
> In the car, on the way home, my father cries. 'I am dying,' he says, 'of this Alzheimer's! I want a cigarette.'
> 'It isn't fatal, Daddy. You could live a long time. You will just forget things.'
> 'That's the same thing as being dead,' he says.
> I reach across the car and put my hand on Daddy's. Staring out the window at the white hills, without turning toward me he clutches my wrist with his hand, cold and

damp with fear. He holds fast, even when I have to shift gears. He holds my hand until we get home, as if letting go would mean spinning away faster into a forgetting place neither one of us can bear to see him go.

(Cohen 2003: 120–1)

Cohen's account illustrates that thoughts about the future are an aspect of these people's experiences of living with dementia (see MacQuarrie 2005). The experience of having dementia both imposes an element of finitude on a person's life and changes the nature of the present. This is seen and experienced in different ways. Perceiving the future as a nightmare with the prospect of a living death is not uncommon (Phinney and Chesla 2003). One response to this fear is a reluctance to looking to the future. Raushi describes this with respect to his illness: 'I cannot live with all of my future life filling today's space. This would be way too heavy a load, and most likely destructive' (Raushi 2004: 108).

However, by the time the future and what it impends is more real and imminent, the person with dementia may no longer be able to verbally articulate their experiences and thoughts.[4] We cited Moniz-Cook et al. (2006) on what people think will happen to them from early in their dementia journey and will return to these concerns in Chapter 6.

For some people a process of seeking to make sense of the changes occurring in their lives prompts an engagement with questions of meaning. These questions relate to wider personal beliefs and values about what it means to be human, about self and about their relationships with others. Whilst often framed in terms of spiritual and religious domains (Boden 1998; Davis 1989), meaning-making is broader, also incorporating psychological and social dimensions.

The processes of adjustment and sense-making are often small scale and iterative (Cheston and Bender 1999; Kitwood 1990), and occur in the daily life-worlds we have described. There are ongoing cycles of response, and adjustment, to the changes and losses the person with dementia encounters, which have been mapped out by Goldsmith (2004). Elements of awareness, recognition, anxiety, depression, assessment and professional 'naming' of the changes, acceptance and understanding of what is happening are identified. These elements create spirals of experience and response which overlap and compound each other.

....

4 The reluctance to adopt a future orientation is evident in many people diagnosed with a life limiting illness. See Small and Rhodes (2000) on this phenomena motor neurone disease, multiple sclerosis and cystic fibrosis.

MacQuarrie (2005) and Clare (2002a, b, 2003) have investigated how people adjust to living with dementia early on in the condition. MacQuarrie (2005) concludes from his conversations with 13 people recently diagnosed with dementia that people engage in paradoxical coping. On the one hand, they acknowledge what is happening to them and on the other actively resist it. MacQuarrie (2005) describes how people accept the disease and its symptoms, express feelings about it, and describe strategies they are using to cope with it while at the same time resisting it through denial, minimization, normalization and reminiscing about former achievements and competence.

Clare (2002a, 2003) studied 12 people in the early stages of dementia. From her conversations she concludes that people demonstrate awareness of changes in cognitive functioning and that they differ both in terms of what these mean for them, and in how they react to them. She describes people's reactions as falling along a continuum of what she calls 'self maintaining' and 'self adjusting'. She describes self-maintaining strategies as those that serve to normalize or minimize changes thus seeking to maintain continuity with the person's prior sense of self. Self-adjusting strategies, on the other hand, serve to integrate the changes into one's conception of oneself. These strategies include confrontation of the change, with a view to adapting one's sense of self to include these changes.

David (in Noyes 2004) describes how he has moved on in his understanding of living and dying with dementia and is able to accommodate both the losses and ensuing grief by living in the present and, as he describes it, 'picking them flowers':

> In the first year or two I was more concerned about thoughts about death. I'm going to miss my daughter's marriage, one way or the other I'm not going to be around for life events. It's a source of grief and loss. There's lots of fear around the unknown. The 'I know how to do this' days are going to go. What's been surprising is getting back to my optimistic side. If you told me two years ago what would happen, stop speaking, stop driving, stop reading … what kind of a fucking life is that? You've taken all my joys! But you know, out of the unknown, the unexpected good things come up. It's easy to focus on the things that have gone but there's no way of knowing what the new things are that are coming. If I can let go, let it flow and not get too attached and tied up, the more I am open to whatever is happening.

> David, in Noyes (2004: 96)

People with dementia may choose to actively engage with their illness and the experiences it brings, or they may not. How, and whether, they do this may reflect their beliefs and values, often drawn from spiritual or religious sources. Bryden (2005) recounts how she has made sense, and found meaning, in her living with dementia. However, this has taken place over a number of years. In her first book, Boden (1998), asks *'Who Will I Be When I Die?'* raising questions of self and identity. Eight years later, she has come to a point of being able to tell her story and know who she is, as a person with dementia thinking about her own mortality. Davis (1989), too, describes the meaning he makes of his journey with Alzheimer's dementia in the context of his Christian faith. He describes a combination of a 'mountain top experience that drew me as close as I have ever been to the sunshine of Christ' and the 'blackest times, in which there was never any moonlight' (Davis 1989: 20).

Other sources of spiritual meaning are described by Morris Friedell:

> Like many persons facing catastrophic illness I've found spirituality helpful. Liberal Judaism teaches that no matter how difficult my situation I can aspire to be a 'mensch', a responsible person who also knows how to enjoy life and is interestingly individual. Buddhism teaches that, whatever my suffering, 'this too shall pass,' and that the dreaded 'loss of self' is, to a significant extent, the mere shedding of illusion.
>
> http://members.aol.com/MorrisFF, downloaded 18 August 2006

However, as people experience greater impairment because of their dementia, their ability to verbally articulate the meaning they make of their circumstances becomes more restricted. Ann Lewin (2006), in a poem written about her mother, reminds us that there are still episodes of lucidity in which a person's understanding of their situation and their forthcoming death, may be communicated.

Still growing

My mother died some time ago.
The person I now care for,
Though she looks the same,
Has lost her power.
No longer archetypal,
Giver of life, solver of problems,
Source of wisdom, but
A frail old lady, confused and
Almost past the stage of knowing it.
(Though suddenly the other night
She said, 'Old age defeats me,
Who'd have thought that I'd go
Funny in the head like this?')

Watching her tears me inwardly.
Why should she suffer this disintegration,
Going on wearily from day to day?

Yet in her waiting there is hope.
Delightful still in personality,
She grows serenely on to her next stage.
Faltering strength and ceasing to be mother
Are staging posts, not ends, for her.
She's waiting in anticipation for her next
Adventure. 'When the time is right,' she says,
'I'll go.'

(Lewin 2004: 103)

Family and friends

The varied nature of the experiences encountered by family members (and friends who are significant to the person with dementia) reflects the diversity of this group of people. Differences in experience arise from their demographic and social status as well as each family's unique dynamics (Nolan *et al.* 2001; Zarit *et al.* 1985; Twigg and Atkin 1994). Family members can be of the same generation as the person with dementia (spouses, partners or siblings), the next adult generation down (children, nephews and nieces) or even grandchildren. For younger people with dementia, the family member may be a parent, or it may be a child. Family members may also have their own particular health conditions that impact on their ability to provide care. They may also have care responsibilities for other people as well as for the person with dementia.

Family members are often important providers of care to people with dementia all the way to the person's death. They take on many roles and these different roles will impact both on themselves and the care that the person with dementia receives. The nature of the care provided is influenced by pragmatic factors such as the distance from the person with dementia. The care given by a family member may be primary care, undertaking directly personal care tasks or secondary care, visiting and supporting other family members providing direct care. The caring roles adopted by different family members are affected by the emotional distance and type of relationships between family members, the dynamics may not be harmonious in relation to the person with dementia or within the wider family. The complexity of family life with divorce, deaths, remarriages, stepchildren, and half siblings can mean that the negotiation around caring roles in the family is often not straightforward.

Some aspects of the experience of family members during their journey have been well documented (Aneshensel *et al.* 1995; Marriott 2003; Nolan *et al.* 1996, 2001; Twigg and Atkin 1994; Zarit *et al.* 1985). This literature has described families as encountering a range of experiences (Zarit *et al.* 1985) including role overload, hassles and a shrinkage of their social world. But there are also positive experiences (Nolan *et al.* 1996) including the emergence of a new closeness. There are characteristically many different demands; people are pulled in all directions. Knowledge about carers' experience specifically with respect to, and at the end-of-life, is more limited (Zarit and Gaugler 2006).

At the start of a long dementia journey it may be family and friends who are first able to observe and articulate changes that are happening around the person with dementia, as described by this daughter.

> We first began to suspect that there was something wrong 22 years ago when my mother seemed very forgetful. Nothing major, just annoying little things. But we knew my father was worried about her. I wasn't particularly worried myself (I guess I thought he was exaggerating) until she invited us for tea. One of her main pleasures had been cooking and she had been very good at it, but the cake she had made for us was only half cooked.
>
> Gillian Bailey (Alzheimer's Society 2003: 11)

These small changes can often be seen and experienced by others before they are recognized as being of any significance by the person with dementia.

Some of the diversity of the family experience is described in fictional and biographical accounts. In Margaret Forster's novel '*Have the Men Had Enough?*' (1989) the story of the final years and months of Grandma's life is recounted. Part of a close-knit family now living in London, the dynamics of past and present are played out in the crucible of her journey from life to death while living with dementia. The story is told from two perspectives, that of the daughter-in-law and the granddaughter.

A key theme in the story concerns the way that the men in her life have had enough of providing care for her. Of her three children, Stuart, the oldest, has decided to have no more to do with the care of his mother. The middle daughter, Bridget, who never married and lives in the next door flat to her mother provides most of the practical care, and Charlie, the youngest son, married to Jenny with two children (Hannah and Adrian), pays for the care that is provided by day carers while Bridget works, and night sitters for the nights Bridget has off. Charlie feels particularly that it is time for his mother to move into a setting where care can be provided all the time. His sister Bridget is adamantly against this and, to a lesser extent, so is his wife.

Present in this story is the complexity of care provision by family members: the numbers of people involved, what happens when something goes wrong, or the pattern is changed (such as one family member going away for a night, or on holiday). Alongside this is the slow but inexorable decline of Grandma, whose language ability alters as does her physical ability to walk and undertake her own daily activities. Many changes are described in her social circumstances.

Initially, Grandma lives in a flat next door to her daughter, Bridget, who provides care for her. Two nights a week a paid carer sits in to give Bridget a break. During the day another carer comes and other members of the family also provide care. The different settings in which Grandma finds herself are described. The day centre she has to leave because of being incontinent and because of how the centre staff perceive her behaviour, the nursing homes to which she gains admission and which she leaves after only three days. She is asked to leave the hospital because nothing is deemed to be wrong with her. Moving into a nursing home is seen by the family to be a major step and, in delaying the move, her condition becomes too advanced to enable her to be accepted into the home and she ends up in a long stay psychogeriatric ward, where she finally dies.

In contrast to Margaret Forster's fictional account, we hear in Federica Caracciolo's (2006) autobiographical account from Italy, her journey alongside her husband (Francesco). She describes a period of seven years from his diagnosis to his death with dementia. The title 'Alzheimer: A Journey Together' captures the core narrative of this book. The notion of journeys and travelling is present in a number of different ways. Travelling abroad to a number of different countries is the wider context in which Federica and Francesco lived their lives: he as an architect and she as a translator. In this account there is a gradual closing down of their lives and the nature of their journeying. This begins with the curtailment of holidays and continues to the difficulties of leaving home to visit friends and familiar places. The final journey Francesco makes to the Villa Flavia (a nursing home) is a relatively brief one and marks the last stage of his life. Different journeys are described as Francesco's illness advances. His decline is charted in the increasing difficulties he has in being physically independent and how these ongoing losses, small and large, impact on his character and appearance, and on their relationship and living arrangements.

As Francesco is less able to communicate verbally, the journeying becomes more internal for Federica. She talks about her loneliness, as relationships outside their marriage are more difficult to sustain. The role of paid carers who live with them in their apartment becomes more important and this impacts on their home, as their presence is both a support and an intrusion in their lives. The wider community in which they are living is present as a practical support and a source of commentary on Francesco's illness, although there is little mention of wider family and their place in this unfolding journey. Despite the losses and the curtailment of their previous lives, Federica describes moments and instances of engagement between them and with others that provide meaning and sustenance during this time. For her, love and her relationship with her husband, help her make sense of the 'backward road' she describes herself as being on.

Present in these accounts, fiction and non-fiction, is the journey with its many dimensions. Four interwoven elements seen in family dementia journeys are the family member's experiences of communication, changing roles, decision-making and meaning-making. Family members, too, are engaged on a journey about 'self' as they engage with numerous changes and adjustments.

We have described earlier in the chapter experiences of communication for the person with dementia, as perceived by family member. Also present in these accounts was the experience of the son and daughter, with the challenges they faced in communicating with their mother. Engagement with a person with dementia, especially when verbal communication is compromised, does not always come easily for family members. As this son describes, he needs to prepare for his time with his mother. When he does this he reaches a meaningful place with her. Such times have hidden rewards.

> As I've played a lot of football in my younger years I know all about mental preparation for games. And I realized early on when visiting my mum that my time there was more productive if I took the time, and effort, to prepare myself mentally beforehand.
>
> I quickly realized that visiting my mum was a lot different than going to an ordinary hospital to visit someone. In the latter instance the biggest factor was making the effort to get there. Your time in the hospital was usually the easy part as the patient could usually converse normally with you and you'd both be energized by the interaction. Also those visits tended to be a lot shorter than the one with my mum.
>
> On the days that I was really up for my visits I could sense that both me and my mum had a sort of spiritual sense of well-being, which surpassed any words. Selflessly concentrating on her ... which again took great discipline as my mind wanders a lot ... also enhanced those visits.
>
> Declan Downs

In thinking about family roles, the provision of care by family members to a person with dementia may occur through choice or may occur because of the existence of assumed roles within a family. This is illustrated in '*Have the Men Had Enough?*' Here, as we described above, the daughter chooses to care for her mother at home, a decision which leads to the daughter-in-law deciding to support this situation, against her own wishes.

The term 'family carer' is often used to describe the family of a person with dementia. However it is a contested term (Twigg and Atkin 1994; Jett 2006). The term family carer could be assigned in recognition of the contribution that a person makes to supporting people with dementia, and/or it could represent a professional defining someone in a way that diminishes and objectifies them. The daughter of a woman with dementia who describes herself as accompanying her mother rather than being a carer illustrates a distinction between what she sees herself doing and, for her, an outsider's definition:

> I don't consider myself primarily a caregiver to a parent with dementia, Alzheimer's or not. I identify myself as my mother's companion. She asked me to accompany her through her last years in 1993. I assented. I also identify myself as my mother's care-giver and 'a caregiver to an Ancient One'. At least as often as I talk about taking care of her, I talk about accompanying her. I more often talk about *the journey* I'm on with my mother rather than the task of taking care of her.
>
> http://themomandmejournals.net/archives/2006_08_20_archive.html#once,
> downloaded 24 August 2006

We develop a similar distinction to that between accompanying and caring when we focus on the difference between 'being with' and 'doing for' in Chapter 6.

The transitions required in the move into a new care setting are particularly significant for family members who have been providing care for the person with dementia at home. A shift to care outside the home may occur on a daily basis, for short periods of respite care, or for a longer term. The ability to care for a person with dementia at home until they die requires a particular set of social, economic, physical and emotional resources (Zarit and Gaugler 2006). When these resources are not combined it is likely that, at some point, the person with dementia will move into a long-term care setting. Whilst no longer providing daily intimate care may be a relief for family members in terms of its physical demands, there may be a period of adjustment to allowing care staff in a long-term care setting to do this care instead (Garity 2006) and a renegotiation of roles and ways in which intimate care can still be given to a loved one (Davies and Nolan 2003; Woods *et al.* 2007).

Another important element of the everyday living experience for family members is the ongoing choices and decisions that have to be made through-out the course of the illness (Hughes and Baldwin 2006; Baldwin *et al.* 2005; Baldwin 2006b). Decisions are often made in the context of an extended period of emotional burden and guilt and can range from decisions about the minutiae of daily living to more fundamental decisions about treatments and care interventions (Potkins *et al.* 2000), as we saw in Federica Caracciolo's description earlier.

The types of decisions family members make, particularly at the end of life (Forbes *et al.* 2000), is influenced by their understandings of dementia as a terminal illness. Whilst the presence of dementia in a person's life may be associated for some people with a 'living death' (Woods 1989), family members are not always able to recognize that the changes in the person with dementia's condition indicate that the person is dying.

In terms of making sense of their experiences of being alongside a person with dementia, family members engage with different aspects of meaning making through the journey. The loss of a caring role, mentioned earlier, is an adjustment family members encounter, as Ann Lewin describes in her poem 'A time to mourn'.

A time to mourn

I have been years grieving
Many little deaths:
Loss of mother, as
The roles reversed and
I became her carer;
Loss of recognition, as
Generations mingled and I
Found myself her mother, sister,
Or, more painful, stranger;
Loss of reference points,
As times and seasons merged
Into long twilight,

And now, her care entrusted
To the hands of others,
Loss of shared experience
Leaves me at a loss.

(Lewin 2004: 106)

Different responses to the approach of the death of the person with dementia are identified. Some family members lack awareness of, or are unable to acknowledge, the process of dying. (Forbes *et al.* 2000; Albinsson and Strang 2003a, b; Collins *et al.* 1993). The future death of their relative is something that some family members do think about, as this granddaughter recounts.

Caring for Grandma always makes me think about her death. When I stay overnight with her, I mount the stairs in the morning to wake her up imagining if I might find a dead body instead of a grandmother in the bed. It would be terrible and it would be a terrible relief. I must correct myself: It *will* be terrible when it happens in the coming months or years. And it *will* be a terrible relief.

(Halling 2004: 131)

The death of a person with dementia has been described by family members as both a tragedy and a blessing (Forbes *et al.* 2000). Other writers have identified the sense of relief that is present when a person with dementia dies (Schulz *et al.* 2003; Collins *et al.* 1993). There may be some variation in reaction that is influenced by cultural affiliation. For example, cultural differences between white and African-American family members have been reported (Owen *et al.* 2001).

The extent to which family members can engage with the person with dementia before they died is seen as an important aspect shaping the experience of their death. This engagement is not necessarily about verbal communication, what is important is the perception that a connection was established before the person with dementia died, as is described by this daughter.

> During the course of the night each of us spent time with Dad individually. As we held him and thanked him for being such a wonderful husband or father to us, we found that the fear and dread left us. It was then that we all started to sense something very special happening. As Dad held each of our hands in turn and kissed us, he maintained intense eye contact and seemed to almost drink our love for him. Each of us sensed this was a mutual exchange. Dad seemed to be giving us something of him-self, a parting gift.

> (Weathers 2002–2003)

Lane (1998), a theologian, describes making sense of his mother's dying. Drawing on biblical imagery he describes a slow, friendly and 'ordinary' death:

> Such were the lessons I began to learn in my frequent visits to the nursing home. When my mother's condition levelled out and even improved in certain ways, I had to rethink the meaning I'd sought from her death. Her own acceptance of death's delay made me reconsider my restless impatience. No longer could I picture myself in tragic terms, defiantly confronting death, eager to get it over with as soon as possible. Instead, a more insistent question began to emerge. How would I cope with the uneventful, living from day to day in the absence of spectacular drama? Finding myself on the slow path to Canaan, I moved through a weary landscape strewn with ostriches and dragons (Lamentations 4:3).
>
> Only in time spent pushing a wheel chair, changing diapers, sitting through long periods of silence, and waiting for nothing can one learn the truths of ordinariness. Life is not a matter of running away from fears, denying the monstrous feelings that lie within us. Life cannot be 'fixed', at least not in the compulsive and controlling way I'd often attempted. There was no cure for my mother or myself, I learned. Healing maybe, but no cure. We both were terminal cases. I even learned that I didn't need her constant approval, although I'd always sought it. My mother's approval didn't come much anymore, and maybe our relationship was cleaner and more honest as a result. All these truths offered by the dragons of the ordinary are as simple as those Robert Fulghrum learned in the kindergarten. They speak of slow and courageous acts of letting go.
>
> There are graces, we all come to realize, that we'd rather not receive. Theologians distinguish between special grace and common grace, but we've never much valued

the latter. Special grace is extraordinary; it comes with drama and flair. We are rescued, singled out in a momentous act of boldness. But common grace falls upon the just and unjust alike. It strikes us as simply too … ordinary.

(Lane 1998: 98)

Lane's account moves the meaning making into the ordinary acts of everyday living. It also highlights the nature of dying and death that the majority of people with dementia experience, because as we explore later (Chapter 6), this is not a heroic, 'fighting against the odds' death, it is protracted and unglamorous and ordinary.

Family members are faced with multiple losses (Sanders and Corley 2003) which can be likened to a series of ongoing bereavements. These will precede and possibly extend beyond the physical death of the person with dementia. Losses include the changes to an individual's ability to communicate, changes in how a person presents him/herself, and they are able to relate to others (Collins *et al.* 1993). Forbes *et al.* (2000) proposes that the family members she interviewed describe a disruption to the life story for a person with dementia, which has to be acknowledged and lived with. Consequently, grief is often expressed before the physical death of the person (Collins *et al.* 1993).

For family members, the physical death of their relative is not the end of the dementia journey. The bereavement experience following the bodily death of a person with dementia can be profound, as is described by Federica Caracciolo.

Never could I have imagined the void that Francesco's death would leave in me. It seemed that suddenly all my energy accumulated over the last years had dissipated. It was not only the psychological pain of the loss of a loved one I was experiencing but also a physical sense of amputation. The great undertaking that had given meaning to my life for more than six years was suddenly no more. I had to recreate my life again starting from scratch.

(Caracciolo 2006: 106–7)

Murna Downs also describes here her responses to her mother's physical death.

The times we had together in your room
Just the two of us
With the world shut out
Singing and dancing
That they are over
That you're no longer sitting in your chair
Waiting
Being
Wondering

Talking to yourself
and then, when I'm there,
telling me of the places you've been
The church
Mass,
the shops,
and seeing Eileen or Dad
Are you really not in your room?
You were always there in your room where I could reach you
always there
that you're no longer there
that in the end you slipped away so quietly.

    Murna Downs

In these accounts we have presented experiences from the point of view of the person with dementia and then from the point of view of the family member. This is commonly how people affected by dementia are thought about: the person and his or her family members. More recently this approach has been challenged and the partnership between these parties, rather than the individual experience, has been given more priority. Robinson *et al.* (2005b) advocate a concern with how the couple adjusts to the changes consequent upon the progression of dementia. They are critical of what they see as a separatist approach. They take a family systems perspective to make sense of how nine couples adjusted to living with dementia, in particular their psychological reactions to early losses. Not unlike MacQuarrie (2005), they describe how couples engage in a dynamic process of coping, both confronting and then avoiding the loss they face. This dynamic oscillation is similar to the 'dual process model' of coping with loss, where one goes back and forth between a focus on loss and on restoration in people experiencing bereavement (see, for example, Stroebe *et al.* 1993, 2001). (In Chapter 3 we look in more detail at how the experiences of dying, death and bereavement in dementia can be understood using the established constructs of bereavement scholarship.)

Places on the journey

From the accounts presented above it can be seen that the person with dementia can live in and visit a variety of places on the journey: their own or others' domestic homes, dementia cafés, day care centres, hospitals, sheltered housing, extra-care housing, long-term care settings such as nursing homes, and possibly hospices. The location a person is in greatly shapes their life-world experiences and is a point of intersection between the life-world and the system world. The number and frequency of transitions into different places varies for any individual, but each change brings with it a need for new adjustments.

People with dementia will spend much of their life living in their own homes and engaging with their local community, as they did prior to a diagnosis. This may persist through the whole dementia journey. In the US, it is estimated that 34 per cent of people with Alzheimer's disease are cared for at home in the last 90 days of life and 34 per cent spent over half of their last 90 days of life at home (Steinhardt 1998).

The importance of remaining at home is often mentioned in people's accounts of living with dementia. In Margaret Forster's story we see the way in which family dynamics respond to Grandma's deteriorating condition and the different levels of commitment to keeping Grandma at home. Federica Caracciolo's account is interesting in its lack of other family apart from herself. Paid carers who support her in caring for her husband at home are needed but remain strangers in the Caracciolo home.

Domestic space, but also the wider social spaces, occupied by the person with dementia and family members have been identified as becoming more constricted as a person's dementia progresses (Holst and Hallberg 2003). Whilst living at home, a person with dementia may visit places of care on a daily basis, or for short periods of time, as a therapeutic intervention or to provide respite breaks for the person caring for them.

A move into sheltered housing or assisted living accommodation is likely to reflect a recognition of a need for increased support. Recent work in the provision of care for people with dementia in supported housing indicates that people with dementia can be supported in this setting until they die (Vallelly et al. 2006). However, if the dementia leads to changes in a person's functional ability, to increased emotional distress or behaviours that are difficult for other people living in that setting, or the person is deemed by others to be unsafe, then they are likely to be asked to move elsewhere (Gillick 2006).

Many people with dementia will move into a long-term care setting. This occurs for a number of reasons, including hospitalization for an acute illness, informal carer breakdown or the death of the carer (carers are often elderly), a sense that the demands upon the person providing care at home are becoming overwhelming and concerns for the person with dementia's well-being and safety (Aneshensel et al. 1995). Variously called care homes (UK), nursing homes (US, UK, Scandinavia), residential aged care facilities (Australia), these facilities provide care for frail older people, of whom a high proportion live with a degree of cognitive disability. These facilities are often categorized by the degree of functional impairment of the residents living in them.

This determines the extent and type of care provided. In Australia this distinction is reflected in the terms 'high' and 'low' care, which is similar to the distinction present in the UK where nursing homes (high care) provide nursing care and a different sort of establishment, residential care (low care) provides only personal care.

In the UK, over half of all people with dementia live in care homes (McDonald and Cooper 2007); consequently, a high proportion of residents in care homes live with a degree of dementia. In 1996, 42–48 per cent of residents in a range of care home settings demonstrated mild impairment, and a further 19–44 per cent of residents demonstrated severe impairment (Darton *et al.* 2003). Higher levels of cognitive and functional impairment are to be found in care homes where nursing care is provided. Australia and Sweden have a higher proportion of residents in high care facilities with dementia, 60 per cent (Gibson *et al.* 1999) and 66 per cent (Sandberg *et al.* 1998) respectively, than is evident in the US, where only 50 per cent of residents live with dementia (Magaziner *et al.* 1985). Figures from Australia (Gibson *et al.* 1999) indicate that half of the people with dementia live in such institutional settings, whilst the rest live at home either independently or with family members.

Hospitals, too, can be significant places where people with dementia can be found. With the changing face of acute hospital care, it is less likely that people with dementia will spend extended periods of time in an acute hospital specifically for treatment for their dementia. It is more likely that they will be admitted for an acute episode of illness such as a respiratory or urinary tract infection (Formiga *et al.* 2004). People with dementia being cared for in a hospital setting, where staff often lack knowledge and confidence to engage with them, can be easily cast into the role of being a problem by staff and by other patients (Health Advisory Service 1998). In hospitals, particularly, there is a potential for conflict between different care goals. Professionals may work to different agendas, some seek a cure, others may focus on maximizing the potential of the 'patient' through rehabilitation, and others prefer to emphasize the palliation of symptoms, whether they be physical or behavioural. Levenson (2004) describes the lack of agreement among professionals involved in her mother's care at the end of her life, stressing that there is an alternative construction where 'dying need not become a medical event' (Levenson 2004: 1244).

The high proportion of people living in long-term care settings means that these places are also likely to be where people with dementia die. In the USA, the majority of older people (67 per cent) whose underlying cause of death is attributable to dementia die in institutional long-term care, in nursing homes (Mitchell *et al.* 2005). In the UK 43 per cent of people with dementia lived (and 41 per cent died) in care homes in the last year of life (McCarthy *et al.* 1997).

Older people with dementia are also more likely to die in hospital than at home, with high rates of hospitalization from care homes noted (Porell 2005). These admissions to hospital prior to death are often short-term and can happen imminently before a person dies, creating added confusion for the person with dementia, their family carers and the receiving staff, who do not know the person. The end of life care provided in these different settings is described in more detail in Chapter 3.

We note that hospices are generally absent in discussions about place for people with dementia, for reasons we discuss in Chapter 6. As we describe in Chapter 3, hospice and specialist palliative care services have sought to address the provision of care for people with dementia.

The life-world in context

In this chapter we have presented a largely subjective account of the life-world for people with dementia and their family carers. In the latter sections we have begun to identify the way in which people's life-worlds are shaped by interactions with the system world. Three key features of the journeys we have described with particular relevance for this life-world/system world juxtaposition are noted here. First, a person with dementia experiences ongoing changes of place of care. Second, there are significant points when interaction between people's life-worlds and the system world is more pronounced: these typically are diagnosis, the use of care services and around the very end of life. Third, what we hear about people's experiences of care is often a story of inconsistent provision. Characteristically either too little or too much is provided.

Prior to diagnosis, engagement with services may be focused on issues of functional ability, cognition, or altered behaviour. The use of day care services or respite services for short periods often precedes a move to a long-term care setting. Increased formal care support in the home may enable a family member or other carer to support a person with dementia at home until they die, but in some instances, a move to a long-term care setting occurs. The bodily death of the person with dementia leads to a final transition for the family members. The way in which formal care service provision addresses the needs of people with dementia and their families will be described in Chapter 3, we then identify the way in which a search for quality has shaped the nature of these services in Chapter 5.

Experiences of care: too little and too much

Implicit in the experiences we have presented are judgements about the quality of care. Whilst we have identified accounts where people with dementia and family have experienced positive things, often during these journeys experiences are described as being less than optimal. Negative aspects of people's experiences are related both to the consequences of the illness upon people's lives, abilities and functioning, but also with respect to their experiences of the care and services that are provided to support them. Present in people's accounts is a paradox of care provision being seen as either too little or too much.

Examples of too little care are seen in terms of the support provided to family carers (Clarke 1999). People from ethnic minorities may be further disadvantaged because of assumptions made by service providers about the availability of family support (Bowes and Wilkinson 2003). In hospitals, examples of deficits in terms of specific interventions for particular symptoms, for example pain (Robinson *et al.* 2005a, Scherder *et al.* 2005) have been identified. There are also differences in terms of the provision of palliative care interventions noted between people with dementia and people without dementia in hospital (Sampson *et al.* 2006). Research from the US suggests that their nursing homes have neither suitable physical environments nor staffing arrangements to ensure quality end of life care (Kayser-Jones 2002; Kayser-Jones *et al.* 2003). There can be a lack of privacy and too much noise. Basic physical care including bathing, oral hygiene, fluids and food intake, and repositioning are suboptimal. Inadequate staffing patterns often exist. There is evidence that in some UK nursing homes interpersonal and psychosocial aspects of care for people with dementia may be limited (Ballard *et al.* 2001a, b). Some of what we have described with respect to too little being provided for people with dementia is not unique to this group of people. Too little, with regard to when issues are addressed and the need to wait for services and help to be provided, is an experience common to many older and disabled people.

With respect to too much, a significant percentage of people with end-stage dementia are administered systemic antibiotics despite their limited utility and potential for generating discomfort (Evers *et al.* 2002). Particularly in the US, many people have nasogastric feeding tubes inserted despite evidence that they neither prolong life nor prevent aspiration in this group, while they do cause discomfort (Gillick 2000). Towards the end of a person's life there may also be inappropriate hospital admissions that do not enhance their experience of care and quality of life (Lamberg *et al.* 2005). The extent to which people are hospitalized as well as how often they change care settings may not be helpful for people with dementia who become easily confused and disorientated without their familiar social and environmental cues. The experience prior to death for many people with dementia who are admitted to hospital is one of an interventionist regime including tube feeding, laboratory tests, the use of restraints, and intravenous medications. The result is not good-quality care even when defined within a narrow medical paradigm. There is evidence of pressure ulcers, constipation, shortness of breath and pain (Mitchell *et al.* 2004). One specific finding in a New York study was that 51 per cent of patients with advanced dementia received a new feeding tube during a terminal hospitalization compared with 11 per cent of patients with metastatic cancer.

> This widespread practice of tube feeding in end-stage dementia is concerning amid growing empirical data and expert opinion that the intervention has no demonstrable health benefits in this population and may be associated with undesirable outcomes, such as the use of restraints.
>
> (Mitchell *et al.* 2004: 325)

As we describe in Chapter 3, there are examples of innovative practice in long-term care settings, but universal good-quality care has not yet been achieved. These issues of too little and too much are symptomatic, we argue later, of a wider dis-ease that society has with dying, and with forms of dying such as dementia that impact on personhood (see Chapters 4 and 6).

Conclusions

The presence of dementia for an individual has profound implications for their living and dying. The ongoing changes that arise from dementia for individuals are both influenced, and influence, how people, services and society engage with the condition and the person who lives with the condition. The long journey has both negative and positive threads running through it, and the extent to which the experience is perceived to be good or bad varies over time and between individuals. It will always be a hard journey because of the multitude of ways dementia impacts on a person's life: cognitively, functionally, emotionally, spiritually, and socially.

In this chapter we began by emphasizing subjective accounts of living and dying with dementia. Given the practical and ethical difficulties of engaging with people with dementia and people who are dying, the accounts have been drawn from people with dementia who are still able to communicate verbally. In addition, we have drawn from the worlds of people with dementia that have been written in poems and family members' accounts. In our emphasis on the importance of place in understanding people's life world, we changed the tone of the chapter. Particular experiences of care need to be located in the wider context of service provision, that is in the system world, and this different tone is present here. This leads us to consider further, in the next chapter, the wider system within which the person with dementia and their family members are situated. The system world is focused around organizational and institutional structures and places (Habermas 1984, 1987). We describe how different discourses exist for health and social care professionals and how the assumptions and priorities of each discourse can change the way in which people's life-world journeys are understood, managed, and experienced.

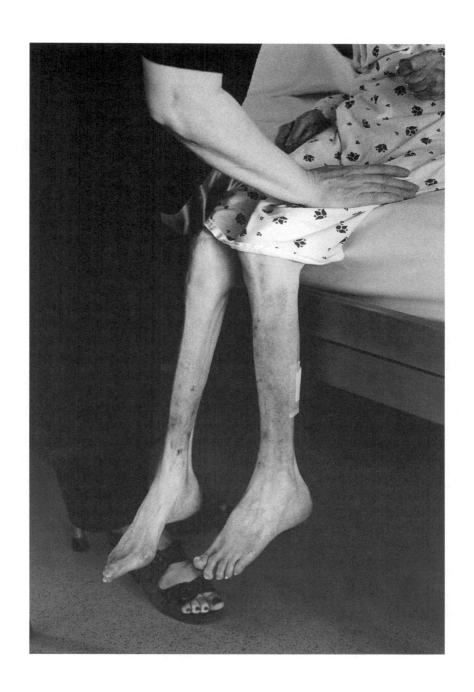

Chapter 3

The system world:
Developments in service provision

When a lot of remedies are suggested for a disease, that
means it can't be cured.
Gaev in (Anton Chekhov, The Cherry Orchard 1917:
Act 2)

Introduction

In Western societies we have established complex organizations and systems
whose purpose is to provide care and support for people with identified
impairments. Caring for frail older people is described as being the 'core business'
of health and social care by Ian Philp in the report *A new ambition for old age:
Next steps in implementing the National Service Framework for Older People*
(Department of Health 2006a: 3).

This chapter is structured around distinctions made in the system world
between care for people with dementia and care for people who are dying. The
chapter argues that it is timely to bring both approaches together.

In the first part of the chapter we examine two key discourses in developing
care for people with dementia and their families: that of clinical medicine and
person-centred care. We note that these key influences in dementia care, while
advocating for the need to address care for people at the end of life, are only
beginning to articulate in detail what this care should comprise. In the second
part of the chapter we go on to consider the development of care for people who
are dying, and explore the challenges that mainstream hospice and palliative care
services face in caring for people with dementia. In the third part of the chapter we
present examples of innovative practices and initiatives from around the world
in palliative care for people with dementia who are dying. We use these as illustrations of how we can work within current systems and structures to engage
with the life world of the person with dementia and that of his or her family
members. We note that these new initiatives are few in number and focused
on specific aspects of the needs of people dying with dementia. We identify

similarities between developments in care for people with dementia and care for people who are dying that have the potential to lead to further innovative work. We will conclude this section by looking at one area that has developed alongside hospice and palliative care, which is the understanding of bereavement and loss. We will consider the ways the insights of this new understanding can link with care of people with dementia.

Throughout the chapter we will see that both segregation and shortcomings in services provided have been the subject of critical attention by those concerned both with care of people with dementia and care for those dying. The need for reform has been prompted by an accumulation of critical reactions to what was in place. Developments in both clinical medicine and person-centred care have led to alternative possibilities for care of people with dementia, just as developments in palliative care improved care for people who are dying. In this chapter we see how people advocating for things to change, and demonstrating that things could be done differently, have spurred the development of alternative approaches to care.

Care for people with dementia

Care and services for people with dementia and their families has seen significant development since the 1970s. Prior to this time dementia was viewed as an inevitable consequence of ageing (Roth 1955) and the predominant service available was 'warehousing' in public institutions (Townsend 1962). While qualitative distinctions between ageing and dementia are not universally accepted (see for example, Bender 2003; Gubrium 1986; Kitwood 1997a), in Western medicine dementia is now considered as distinct from ageing. For almost 30 years arguments have been made that care needs to address the needs of people with dementia and their families through diagnosis to death and bereavement (Arie 1977; Pitt 1974). Despite this, it is well recognized that such care is not consistently available (Audit Commission 2000) and is in need of an agreed standard (Burns 2005).

In the UK, the National Institute for Health and Clinical Excellence and the Social Care Institute for Excellence (2006) have produced guidance for such care, *Dementia: supporting people with dementia and their carers in health and social care*. This follows the Audit Commission (2000) report *Forget-me-not* detailing the variability of health and social care provision for older people with mental health problems, updated in 2002. The Department of Health's (2001a) *National Service Framework for Older People* outlines a strategic plan with a methodology for performance measurement for reform of health and social care services, setting national standards of care and defining service models. The European Dementia Consensus Network (EDCON) (Burns 2005) has recommended the development and application of quality standards for different types of care throughout Europe, stressing that they take the perspective of people with dementia and their families in to account. (Chapter 5 specifically examines quality standards.)

The development of care for people with dementia and their families can be traced through the history of advocacy by family members (see Fox 2000 and Zarit 2006 for an overview), innovative practitioners and diverse professional groups. In our consideration of the development of care for people with dementia we focus on the efforts of clinical medicine as one of the dominant system views on dementia – particularly geriatric medicine, old age psychiatry, and geriatric neuropsychiatry – and the guiding principles and practices of the person-centred approach to care. In so doing we recognize we are omitting from our discussion the influence on service development from areas within clinical psychology (Woods and Britton 1977; Woods and Clare 2007), nursing (Keady *et al.* 2003, in press) social work (Marshall and Tibbs 2006), and people with dementia themselves (Bartlett and O'Conner, 2007).

Clinical medicine

In the UK the specialities of geriatric medicine and old age psychiatry have influenced the development of care for people with dementia. Perhaps more influential in the US, geriatric neuropsychiatry has also influenced approaches to care. As we will see, to a lesser or greater extent, these world views see the person in terms of 'symptoms' which need to be 'managed'.

Geriatric medicine

Geriatric medicine, as a specialty, grew out of the recognition that it was possible to treat, or minimize the disabling effects of, many health problems of old age. Geriatric medicine has as its aim improving health for older people. The strap line for the British Geriatrics Society is 'for health in old age' (www.bgs.org.uk, accessed 3 February 2007), while the strap line for the American Geriatrics Society is 'dedicated to the health of older Americans' (www.americangeriatrics.org, accessed 3 February 2007). From the web site of the British Geriatrics Society we can see that

> Geriatric Medicine (Geriatrics) is that branch of general medicine concerned with the clinical, preventive, remedial and social aspects of illness in older people. Their high morbidity rates, different patterns of disease presentation, slower response to treatment and requirements for social support call for special medical skills.

The purpose is to restore an ill and disabled person to a level of maximum ability and wherever possible return the person to an independent life at home.

In this section we will argue that this emphasis on restoration and maximization of function risks excluding people with dementia and others who live with progressive and chronic conditions.

When the UK National Health Service was established in 1948 the prevalent view was that sickness in old age could not be cured or treated: custodial care was all that could be provided to older people living with chronic conditions. People in this category, particularly those who were poor, were accommodated, most commonly, in local authority hospitals (often old Poor Law infirmaries). Townsend (1962) referred to such accommodation as 'warehousing'. There was then 'a predominantly segregated service where old, frail individuals could at best expect benign guardianship until they died rather than active treatment aimed at their ultimate discharge, (Jefferys 2000: 76).

This situation was confronted, and changed, particularly by the work of two superintendents of poor law infirmaries, Marjory Warren and Lionel Cosin. They initiated innovative treatment regimes that included thorough medical examination, diagnosis and rehabilitation programmes for older people, with the result they recovered physical and mental capacities, re-engaged with personal hygiene concerns and with undertaking activities of daily living. Some returned home, some moved into residential care. Warren and Cosin fought against the segregation of older people in the health service and Marjory Warren, in particular, fought to establish the specialty of geriatric medicine (Evers 1993). The Medical Society for the Care of the Elderly was founded in 1947 and this became the British Geriatrics Society in 1959. Marjory Warren combined charisma, great clarity of vision and an ability to marshal committed groups of supporters in the pursuit of a specific goal, over a long period of time in the face of indifference, or hostility, from the medical, health service and care establishment (see Jefferys 2000: 76, 86).

The early initiatives by Warren and Cosin and more recent developments within geriatric medicine have mirrored a more general aspiration in society that seeks to emphasize healthy ageing and the maximization of functional ability for as long as possible. There is however an evident paradox – more and more people are living into old age and this is viewed as a sign of social progress, yet the chronic illnesses of old age that also have become prominent have yet to be adequately addressed (Department of Health, 2001a).

Current geriatric service provision for older people, certainly in the UK, aims to correct problems and ensure the maximization of physical function. The *National Service Framework for Older People* (Department of Health 2001a) recommends support is provided to ensure that older people can stay in their own homes, and promotes the development of intermediate care settings where people can receive intensive support to maximize their abilities and then return home after an acute illness or trauma. As such geriatric medicine has become rehabilitative in focus, supporting older people to regain and then maintain functional ability to maximize the possibilities of their being independent. Despite its earlier inclusion of older people with mental health problems (e.g. Exton-Smith and Evans 1977; Williamson *et al.* 1964), the current emphasis on cure and rehabilitation of the body is pursued at the expense of prioritizing care where cure is not possible, for example attention to mental health issues.

In the US there is a similar emphasis within geriatric medicine on maximizing older people's functional ability. Funding issues are a considerable influence on the form of geriatric service provided. The Medicare system supports an interventionist regime of health care provision (Gillick 2006) and alternative modes of supporting people who have multiple chronic conditions are not easily accommodated in such a system.

The discourse and the service organization of geriatric medicine have consequences for the care of people with dementia. First, the emphasis on physical functioning may not improve quality of living. Gillick (2006) asks if it will lead to fewer years with disability and dependence, compressing morbidity into the very last years of life, or if it will increase the period of frailty for older people. Second, the emphasis on physical ability means that the impact of mental health problems, including cognitive impairment, on quality of life may be underestimated. Third, there is an assumed level of cognitive ability needed for rehabilitation that excludes people whose cognitive abilities have changed. Despite landmark texts calling for an approach to rehabilitation which accommodates the needs and circumstances of people with dementia (e.g. Marshall 2005; Perrin and May 1999), with notable exceptions (e.g. Clare 2002a, b), there is not evidence of a strong rehabilitative ethic in the everyday care of people with dementia. Finally, a focus on cure and rehabilitation within geriatric medicine implies that for people with dementia dying is not, generally, proactively addressed – either at the time of diagnosis or sometimes at the end of life. This leads to their dying not being well managed. The fragmented approach to service provision leaves the person at risk of experiencing a lot of change and disruption in the last years and months of life, perhaps separated from sustaining relationships and social support. Despite this having been a concern for at least 20 years (e.g. Volicer 1986), it has yet to be adequately addressed.

Old age psychiatry

In the UK old age psychiatry, also referred to as psychogeriatrics, developed in the late 1960s to assess, treat and manage mental health problems experienced by older people living both in the community and in institutional settings. The specialty grew from the recognition by psychiatrists that a significant percentage of their clients were older people and from geriatricians that a significant number of their patients experienced mental health problems, particularly cognitive impairment (Pitt 1974). In the UK old age psychiatry combines a knowledge of drug treatment with a 'psychosocial and psychotherapeutic attitude' (Burns 2001: 185), relying on the use of a broad range of skills and expertise including medicine, particularly social medicine, family dynamics, psychological and neurological testing, and clinical acumen (Pitt 1974). Arie and Jolley (1982) outline the principles of an old age psychiatry service as including home-based assessment and collaboration with others including nurses, social workers, geriatric medicine and primary care practitioners (see Hilton 2005 for an overview).

The 1996 consensus statement on *Psychiatry of the elderly*, jointly produced by the World Health Organization and the Geriatric Psychiatry section of the World Psychiatric Association, identified the key characteristics of old age psychiatry being its community focus and 'multidisciplinary approach to assessment, diagnosis and treatment' (1996: 3). Such an approach recognized that dementia frequently co-occurs with age-associated health problems, sensory impairments and changes in social circumstances. Recognizing the dementias as progressive, the aim of intervention should be promoting quality of life by, amongst other things, emphasizing abilities alongside deficits and attending to the patient's and his/her family's experience. Old age psychiatry stressed the importance of being part of a community-based team conducting assessments in the home and developing care plans which support the person in living in the community (Arie and Isaacs 1977).

Old age psychiatry services have taken the lead in assessment, diagnosis and care for people with dementia (Banerjee 2007) and this model of care has spread to other parts of the world (see Draper *et al.* 2005 for a review). Along with geriatricians (Wilcock *et al.* 1999), old age psychiatrists have played a key role in the development of memory clinics, providing assessment, information, treatment, education, and research. Such clinics have grown in number in the last decade, this growth being in part attributed to the availability of anti-dementia drugs (Lindesay *et al.* 2002) and policy guidance by the Department of Health (2001a). The quality of the service provided is being reviewed (Phipps and O'Brien 2002), alongside the development of an evidence base for their effectiveness in promoting quality of life (Moniz-Cook and Woods 1997).

Despite the long history of concern with older people's mental health and government policy that all areas should have an old age psychiatry service (Banerjee 2007), the variability of service provision is of concern (Audit Commission 2000; Banerjee 2007). Given relatively low provision of the service, those who do have contact with old age psychiatry tend to be those with 'severe and complex disorders where there are high levels of risk and co-morbidity' (Banerjee 2007: 4).

For many people with dementia their only health service contact is with primary care. While some argue that diagnosis of dementia can be conducted in primary care settings, others argue that this should be the domain of old age psychiatry or specialist services (Banerjee 2007). There is, however, widespread agreement that primary care teams have a key role to play in the provision of ongoing support to people with dementia and their families (Department of Health 2001a; National Institute for Health and Clinical Excellence/Social Care Institute for Excellence (NICE/SCIE) 2006). Despite this, many families cite primary care as failing to provide fundamental information and support, while primary care practitioners feel poorly prepared for this role (Audit Commission 2000; Pettit 2000). While educational interventions show some promise in improving practice (Downs et al. 2006a), consumer-directed efforts are increasingly recommended (Ariss et al. 2006).

How the service world responds when someone starts their journey with dementia has been the focus of considerable concern: delayed diagnosis and failure to share the diagnosis is common. This has led the Department of Health (2001a) to focus on this as one of the key areas for development of services in the UK. Sharing the diagnosis has been a vexed issue in the field of dementia care for some time. Until recently the situation was similar to that seen with cancer 50 years ago. Cancer then, and dementia now, can be characterized as a disease where most people dare not speak its name. The benefits and drawbacks to disclosure have been debated since the early 1990s (Drickamer and Lacks 1992). There is now increased evidence that people with dementia want to be told their diagnosis (Pinner and Bouman 2003) and a trend to suggest that, whereas families were once reluctant for their relative to be told (Maguire et al. 1996), this is now less likely to be the case (Pinner and Bouman 2003).

One of the arguments against establishing and disclosing a diagnosis of dementia has been a concern that people with dementia risk experiencing many of the same negative consequences of psychiatric labelling as their younger counterparts (Mackenzie 2006). These include stigma, diagnostic overshadowing and discrimination (Graham et al. 2003). Diagnostic overshadowing results in everything that the person with a diagnosis does or says being attributed to their psychiatric condition (Rosenhan 1973). In this way psychiatric labels have been criticized for leading to consequences which can be as damaging as the effects of the condition itself.

Geriatric neuropsychiatry

Geriatric neuropsychiatry, like old age psychiatry, is concerned with assessment and treatment of psychiatric problems associated with neurological diseases of old age, including dementia. It is an emerging discipline distinguished from old age psychiatry in the degree to which it emphasizes the biological or neurological basis of symptoms. As such, geriatric neuropsychiatry is one of the knowledge bases drawn on by old age psychiatry when caring for an older person with dementia.

Geriatric neuropsychiatry, and neuropsychiatry more broadly, has made several contributions to the advancement of knowledge about dementia through its 'links with basic science and the application of pharmacological treatments to disease and the assessment and management of psychiatric aspects of neurological disease' (Burns 2001: 185). While not without its critics (e.g. Kitwood 1997a; Bender 2003), these include: clarification of the major subtypes of dementia, detailing the behavioural and psychological symptoms of dementia, and applying drug treatments to both cognitive and behavioural and psychological symptoms of dementia.

Neuropsychiatry has made a key contribution to our understanding of the subtypes of dementia. As we described in Chapter 1, dementia is a term used to refer to a syndrome, or collection of symptoms, thought to be caused by a variety of underlying neuropathologies. These underlying neuropathologies are reflected in different patterns of onset, symptoms and patterns of decline (Ballard 2000). The difficulty in establishing the underlying cause of dementia, that is, a differential diagnosis, is well recognized and it is increasingly recognized that many people have mixed underlying pathologies (Ballard 2000). Murphy warns:

> Clinical convention and practice requires us to use a common language but current classification systems will surely become increasingly obsolete as the diverse pathophysiological pathways that result in clinical end-stage overt dementia are identified.
>
> (Murphy 2000: 917)

Existing subtypes of dementia include Alzheimer's disease, vascular dementia, Lewy body dementia and frontotemporal dementia alongside other rarer dementias such as human immunodeficiency virus type 1 associated dementias, dementia associated with alcoholism, and Creutzfeldt-Jakob disease. Alzheimer's disease, considered to be the most commonly occurring underlying neuropathology of dementia, accounts for approximately 60 per cent of those diagnosed with dementia. Progress is gradual, with significant impairment in learning and memory being the most evident early change, leading to impairments in reasoning, planning and organization abilities over time, and ending in severe impairment in almost all cognitive, including language, and motor functions (Forstl 2000).

The different stages of the disease are termed mild, moderate, severe and terminal (Reisberg 1988) and are illustrated in Table 3.1. The stages identified

Table 3.1 Comparison of stages of illness in dementia | 67

Disease stages (1) (Cohan 1997)	Disease stages (2) (Kuhn *et al.* 1997)	Functional Assessment Staging Scale (Reisberg 1988)
Early-stage Memory loss Time and spatial disorientation Poor judgement Personality changes Withdrawal or depression Perceptual disturbances	**Early** Recent memory loss Mild aphasia Seeks familiar and avoids unfamiliar Some difficulty writing and using objects Apathy, depression Needs reminder with some activities of daily living	1. No difficulty either subjectively or objectively. 2. Complaints that locations of objects have been forgotten, subjective work difficulties 3. Decreased job functioning, difficulty in travelling to new locations, decreased organisational capacity.
Mid-stage Recent and remote memory worsens Increased aphasia Apraxia Hyperorality Disorientation to place and time Restlessness or pacing Perseveration Irritability Loss of impulse control	**Middle** Chronic, recent memory loss Moderate aphasia May get lost at times even inside home Repetitive actions, apraxia Possible mood and behavioural disturbances Needs reminders and help with most ADL	4. Decreased ability to perform complex tasks. 5. Required assistance in choosing proper clothing to wear for the day, season or occasion. 6A. Improperly putting on clothes without assistance or cuing occasionally or more frequently over the past weeks. 6B. Unable to bathe properly occasionally or more frequently over the past weeks. 6C. Inability to handle mechanics of toileting occasionally or more frequently over the past weeks.
Late-stage Incontinence of urine or faeces Loss of motor skills, rigidity Decreased appetite and dysphagia Agnosia Apraxia Communication severely impaired May not recognize self or family members Loss of most/all self-care abilities Cognition severely impaired Immune system depressed	**Late** Mixes up past and present Expressive and receptive aphasia Misidentifies familiar persons and places Bradykinesia, at risk for falls Greater incidence of mood and behavioural disturbances Needs help with all ADL Terminal No apparent link to past or present Mute or few incoherent words Oblivious to surroundings Little spontaneous movement, dysphagia, myoclonus, seizures Completely passive Requires total care	6D. Urinary incontinence (occasionally or more frequently over the past weeks). 6E. Faecal incontinence (occasionally or more frequently over the past weeks). 7A. Ability to speak limited to approximately a half-dozen different intelligible words or fewer in the course of an average day or in the course of an intensive interview. 7B. Speech ability limited to the use of a single intelligible word in an average day or in the course of an intensive interview. 7C. Loss of ambulatory ability. 7D. Inability to sit up without assistance. 7E. Loss of ability to smile. 7F. Loss of ability to hold up head independently.

in these approaches are assumed to relate to the degree of support required to maintain a person's living. Mild dementia is where a person retains the ability to manage independently. Moderate dementia requires a person to have a degree of support to maintain independent living and severe dementia results in a situation where the person requires continuous support and help. Different writers describe slightly different stages (Cohan 1997; Kuhn 1997; Reisberg 1988) but, as can be seen in the language used, all focus on symptoms in terms of deficit and dysfunction.

It has been suggested that the stages of progressive loss evidenced in dementia take place in the same orderly sequence as those observed in the attainment of abilities throughout childhood, that is, they can be characterized as 'retrogenesis' (Reisberg 1988). In 2004, Barry Reisberg was awarded a lifetime achievement award from the Alzheimer's Association for his work in this area (Box 3.1):

Box 3.1 The work of Dr Barry Reisberg

In the early 1980s Dr. Reisberg began describing, in many cases for the first time, the precise clinical course of Alzheimer's, which was then largely uncharted territory. His observations ultimately yielded several assessment scales of the stages and symptoms of the disease, the most common form of dementia affecting people over age 65. Over time these scales made it possible for clinicians to identify the specific developmental stages of Alzheimer's patients and to assess their health-care needs. Based on their careful observations, Dr. Reisberg and his colleagues established that the stages of Alzheimer's mimic regression toward infancy: patients lose the ability to hold a job, handle finances, choose clothes, dress and bathe, control their bladder and bowels, and speak – reversing the order in which those skills were acquired as a child. Dr. Reisberg has coined the term 'retrogenesis' to describe the characteristic decline of Alzheimer's patients. He continues to refine his observations of mental and behavioral symptoms, even among normally aging people experiencing occasional forgetfulness, in order to obtain better prognostic markers for the disease. Today, Dr. Reisberg's scales, along with clinical descriptions of the progression of Alzheimer's, are widely used as pivotal measures in determining the efficacy of Alzheimer's disease treatments. The Center for Medicare Services in the United States, as well as some Canadian provinces, have mandated usage of Dr. Reisberg's measures.

From NYU School of Medicine,
http://www.med.nyu.edu/communications/news/pr_60.html, accessed
10 November 2006

Critics question the relevance of stage models for framing the progress of dementia (Bender 2003; Kitwood 1997a). Within the dementia field there are concerns about assuming an inevitability and orderliness of deterioration and questions have been raised about the value of seeking to encapsulate this process in a stage-based model. Furthermore, the uncritical acceptance of the stage approach to conceptualizing dementia captures a resulting dissonance between system world assumptions and the experience of practice and of lived experience or life-world concerns.

There are parallels in palliative care, for example in debates about progression for people with HIV infection. Here, a remorseless shift from HIV positive status, via AIDS-related syndrome to 'full-blown' AIDS was posited early in the epidemic. Critics of stage-based models of decline, in general, questioned how far such formulations reflected day-to-day experience, or helped the people themselves, their carers or the immediate professionals involved in care (Treichler 1992). Rather, these models were understandable as attempts to create social constructions of reality that allowed us, the public and professionals, to contemplate distressing and frightening phenomena in ways that promised *us* a route to understanding and management (see Berger and Luckman 1967).

Vascular dementia is considered to be the second most common cause of dementia, accounting for between 10–50 per cent of people with dementia, depending on geographical location (Erkinjunnti 2000). Unlike Alzheimer's disease, there is a role for prevention in vascular dementia. In Alzheimer's disease the predominant impairments are in memory and language, but people with vascular dementia experience impairments predominantly in executive functioning (processing information, making decisions based on information provided, planning). While change can occur slowly over time, stepwise progression with periods of stability and improvement are also evident (Erkinjunnti 2000). Dementia with Lewy bodies, accounting for approximately 20 per cent of people with dementia, is characterized by progressive and fluctuating cognitive impairment, particularly with respect to attention and visuospatial perception, visual hallucinations and motor impairments (McKeith 2000).

Frontotemporal dementia (FTD), unlike the dementias discussed so far, occurs most commonly in those aged between 45 and 65 (Neary 2000). FTD is so called because of the underlying pathological changes occurring within the frontotemporal lobes of the brain. Unlike other dementias, impairments in cognition are not the predominant feature of FTD, rather, changes in personality and in personal and social conduct along with diminished expressive language predominate (Neary 2000). Other rarer dementias are also more common in younger age groups including human immunodeficiency virus type 1-associated dementias. Traditionally younger people with dementia have been poorly served by the system world (Baldwin *et al.* 2003; Cox and Keady 1998). Recent guidance from the NICE/SCIE (2006) has highlighted the special needs of younger people with dementia and the need for multidisciplinary services for assessment, diagnosis and treatment.

Behavioural and psychological symptoms

From a neuropsychiatric perspective, behavioural and psychological symptoms are viewed as integral, to varying degrees, to many of the diseases underlying dementia. They are referred to as the Behavioural and Psychological Symptoms of Dementia (BPSD) (Finkel *et al.* 1996) and include 'personality alterations, delusions, hallucinations, mood disorders, disorders of neurovegetative (e.g. appetite and sleep) function and troublesome behaviours' (Mirea and Cummings 2000: 61). These psychological and behavioural symptoms are viewed as manifestations of specific underlying pathologies in specific brain regions and, most importantly, as being 'distinct from reactions of the person to their declining abilities' (Mirea and Cummings 2000: 61).

This focus on psychological and behavioural aspects as being neuropsychiatric in origin has been criticized for neglecting the psychological and social aspects of living with dementia (Lyman 1989). In addition, there have been concerns raised that attributing behaviour to underlying neuropathology risks overlooking circumstances when the person with dementia is using behaviour as a form of communication (Snow and Shuster 2006; Stokes 2003). For example, a person may be experiencing pain but lack the requisite language to express this pain (Forstl 2000). When a person is being helped to dress this may accentuate their pain, and they may strike out. If this behaviour is attributed to inevitable symptomatology associated with neuropathology, for example 'troublesome behaviours', either as 'agitation' or 'violence', the person's pain is at risk of being ignored. Given the considerable literature on poor assessment and treatment of pain in people with dementia (eg Cohen-Mansfield and Lipson 2002), this concern is far from trivial.

Drug treatment for cognitive and non-cognitive symptoms

Neuropsychiatry is most commonly associated with the application of drug treatments to the symptoms of dementia – both cognitive and behavioural and psychological symptoms. The availability of medication for the treatment of cognitive symptoms is a relatively recent phenomenon. In the UK, in contrast to earlier guidance, the NICE/SCIE (2006) now recommends the use of three acetylcholine inhibitors (donezepil, galantamine, and rivastigmine) as options in the management of people with Alzheimer's disease of moderate severity. Previous guidance had recommended their use to people in the early stages of Alzheimer's disease. Their prescription must be initiated by a physician specializing in the care of older people and reviewed every six months. Currently no medications are recommended for the treatment of cognitive symptoms for those with any of the other subtypes of dementia. This recommendation is currently being challenged in the high court by the Alzheimer's Society (2007a).

Unlike the relatively recent history of prescribing medication of cognitive symptoms, there has been a long history of the inappropriate use of medication for behavioural symptoms of dementia (Margallo-Lana *et al.* 2001; McGrath and Jackson 1996). There is broad agreement that psychosocial and environmental approaches ought to be the first choice in caring for people with behavioural and psychological symptoms of dementia (Bird 2000; Howard *et al.* 2001; NICE/SCIE 2006). Citing research, Ballard and O'Brien (1999) conclude that neuroleptic medication prescribed for behavioural symptoms has only modest efficacy with high placebo response and is associated with significant side effects, including reduced quality of life. Reduced reliance on psychotropic, including neuroleptic, medication has been achieved by providing psychosocial care (Fossey *et al.* 2007) and appropriate stimulation and activities (Cohen-Mansfield and Werner 1997; Rovner *et al.* 1996).

To summarize, we have made four key arguments in reviewing the role of clinical medicine in the development of services for people with dementia and their families. First, older people with chronic conditions such as dementia have traditionally been underserved by medicine. It is only since the 1950s and 1960s that the specialties of geriatric medicine and old age psychiatry respectively have developed. Secondly, within geriatric medicine the focus on maximizing function and rehabilitation has not been extended to the care of people with dementia. Thirdly, the promise of a well-resourced old age psychiatry service has yet to be realized, despite government rhetoric. Fourth, while useful in furthering our understanding of the underlying neuropathology of the dementias, neuropsychiatry, with its emphasis on drug treatments for cognitive and behavioural symptoms, has had limited influence on the development of services for people with dementia.

Person-centred care

Person-centred is a widely used, yet poorly defined, approach to care for people with dementia (Brooker 2007). The NICE/SCIE (2006) guideline on dementia care has sought to have the principles of person-centred care reflected in its recommendations, recognizing that they underpin best practice in the field. Person-centred care is enshrined as one of the key principles guiding the Department of Health (2001a) *National Service Framework for Older People*.

Person-centred care grew out of disillusionment with the limits of a bio-medical approach to care. Kitwood (1987, 1990, 1996) argued that because medicine was focused almost exclusively on cure, it neglected those whose condition was not amenable to cure. It was this perceived abandonment by the medical profession that provided for Kitwood a moral argument to present an alternative 'process' of dementia – the dialectical model – and an alternative approach to care: person-centred care.

The dialectics of dementia

In Kitwood's (1990, 1996) alternative 'process' of dementia, the 'dialectics of dementia', he challenged the field to consider that neuropathology alone did not account for the changes observed in someone living with dementia. For Kitwood, as for Engel (1977) before him, neuropsychiatric discourse was overly simplistic and deterministic. Consistent with his colleagues in old age psychiatry (e.g. Arie 1970), he argued for a more dynamic and bio-psychosocial view of dementia. This alternative model of dementia argued that change in functioning and quality of life was caused by a dynamic interplay between neurological, psychological and social factors. It is worthy of note that this need to blend medical and social models of health and illness with respect to chronic conditions was formally recognized by the World Health Organization in 2002, and with respect to dementia is advocated by the NICE/SCIE (2006) guidance in the UK.

From a psychological point of view Kitwood stressed two interrelated concepts: that of personhood and that of psychological needs. For Kitwood personhood was essential to optimal functioning. The greatest threat to a person's well-being comes from a potential loss of personhood, or a withdrawal of recognition of their humanity (Kitwood 1993a, b). In the symbolic interactionist tradition of Mead (1932) Kitwood (1990) argued that personhood was created in interaction with others. For Kitwood (1997a: 8) personhood is a 'standing or status that is bestowed upon one human being, by others, in the context of relationship and social being. It implies recognition, respect and trust'. He was interested in documenting the effects of interactions and relationships on people with dementia. Kitwood (1997a) and others (e.g. Lyman 1989, 1998) argued that living with dementia had both psychological[1] and social consequences. Preceding Lyman (1998) and

Post (2000ab)[2], Kitwood argued that it was the threat to personhood that was the greatest threat to a person living with dementia. It was this risk of no longer being viewed as a human being, with all the moral standing this entails, that most threatened the individual. (This is an area further explored in Chapter 4.)

For Kitwood (1997a), people with dementia, like all people, had core psychological needs which if unmet led to distress and dysfunction. These psychological needs included needs for comfort, identity, attachment, occupation, and inclusion. He sought to illustrate the potential for a person with dementia to experience a 'downward spiral' when their personhood and psychological needs were ignored or, even if unintentionally, undermined.

In proposing a role for psychological and social factors in a person's quality of life, Kitwood (1995) introduced a therapeutic optimism into dementia care. For if there were no biological treatments available for the underlying disease, he argued, perhaps it could be arrested or delayed, or at the very least its effects ameliorated, by attending to the psychological and social aspects of a person's life (Downs et al. 2005).

Person-centred care

In proposing person-centred care Kitwood (1995, 1997a) was arguing that care that addressed the psychological and social aspects of living with dementia could slow, if not reverse, much of the deterioration observed. Person-centred care as developed by Kitwood drew on Roger's (1961) work on client-centred psychotherapy, an approach that derived its values from existential phenomenology (Embleton Tudor et al. 2004) and on Buber's notion of the significance of an *I–Thou* mode of relating as opposed to an approach to relating that is built on objectification, hierarchy and difference. These ways of relating are characteristic of the way people with dementia had been approached by service providers, and by members of the public more generally (Buber 1970; see Small et al. 2006). Through providing unconditional positive regard (unconditional acceptance), an empathic understanding (adopting the perspective of the person), and congruence (or being authentic and not aloof) (Rogers 1961) with a person with dementia, therapeutic potential could be realized. Kitwood (1998) referred to relationships and interactions which affirm personhood as 'positive person work'. Such a supportive social psychology incorporates the essence of person-centred care (Brooker 2007, 2004).

Person-centred care was not the only force arguing for a therapeutic approach to people with dementia. At the same time there had been some success in a

Box 3.2 Person-centred care

An approach to caring for people with dementia that seeks to affirm continuing 'personhood' (and that, in so doing, challenges a previously prevalent 'malignant social psychology').

Person-centred care:

- Affirms the value of a person and their life regardless of disability
- Recognizes that people cope actively with dementia
- Seeks to minimize the impact of cognitive, functional and behavioural impairments on a person's quality of life
- Addresses physical, emotional, spiritual and social aspects
- Recognizes the role of life history and personality
- Insists that each person be treated as an individual
- Recognizes that family and staff play a key role in maintaining personhood and quality of life
- Recognizes that family and care staff need support

(Kitwood 1997a)

series of interventions aimed at improving cognition and functioning in the present, most notably using reality orientation (Woods and Britton 1977), demonstrating that people with dementia could still learn from, and participate in, present reality. Woods and Holden's (1982) seminal work *Reality orientation: Psychological approaches to the confused elderly*, was influential in leading to the development of the specialty area of clinical psychology for older people with mental health problems (Woods and Britton 1985). Unlike this work, however, Kitwood did not see improving cognition or orientation as being the main aim of dementia care. Rather, for him, emotional well-being and person-hood were the key indicators of quality of life. Kitwood was keen to pay as much attention to abilities which were left intact as to those which were compromised (Kitwood and Bredin 1992a, b). Brooker (2007) refers to Kitwood's enriched model of dementia.[1] Thus care was not simply about custodial containment for those of no value to society but could be utilized to improve well-being. This enables a member of care staff to have the sense that

---

[1] There were some interesting parallels in laboratory science. Diamond (2001) demonstrated the role of enriched environments in promoting nerve cell growth and the inhibiting effects of impoverished environments in laboratory animals.

there were achievable goals and that care could not just contain but enhance self-actualization and help maintain quality of life.

The person-centred approach in dementia care challenged the inevitability of behavioural and psychological symptoms in dementia, as argued by geri-atric neuropsychiatry. From a person-centred perspective, behaviours, rather than being symptomatic of neuropathology, were, as often, attempts at com-munication and at meeting emotional or social needs (Rader *et al.* 1985; Kitwood 1997a; Stokes 2003). For Jones, 'behaviours exhibited in dementia still express meaning, symbolically if not explicitly' (Jones 1992: 3). Within this approach, behaviours are understood as attempts to communicate and meet needs, be they physical, emotional or social in origin (Beattie *et al.* 2004; Stokes 2003). (See Bird 2000; Bird *et al.* 2002 on ways of understanding behaviour in dementia). This new way of approaching dementia meant there was an assertion of the importance of the personal and social context in which neuro-logical loss takes place (Cheston 1998; Cheston and Bender 1999).

Kitwood, while a charismatic leader and powerful intellectual force in his own right (see Baldwin and Capstick, forthcoming), was part a broader move-ment concerned with the psychological and social aspects of living with dementia taking place throughout the UK and US. He articulated the dissatisfac-tion that many people felt seeing their relatives and clients reduced to a language of deficit and dysfunction. In the United States the dominance of a geriatric neuropsychiatric perspective was challenged by, amongst others, Karen Lyman (1989) and Joanne Rader. Lyman's (1989) seminal paper *Bringing the social back in: critiques of the bio-medicalisation of dementia*, called for a reconsideration of the social factors which affected the quality of life of people with dementia. Rader and colleagues (1985) attributed meaning to the behaviour of people with dementia, describing behaviour that others considered challenging as 'agenda behaviour' or behaviour driven by an attempt to meet a need. Amongst other things, this view has prompted a line of research into needs-related behaviour led by Beattie and colleagues (2004). In Sweden, Astrid Norberg and colleagues were calling for an approach to care for people with dementia who they viewed as being actively engaged in reconciling their lives, however confused their state of mind (Kihlgren *et al.* 1994), leading them to promote 'integrity–promoting care' as that which supported people in their life review work. This interest in people's active engagement in life resolution is also found in Feil's (1982) validation work with people with dementia. Finnema's (2000) emotion-oriented care stressed the importance of attending to emotion in dementia care.

The 1990s saw growth in the therapeutic potential of psychological and social care for people with dementia as indicated in titles such as Holden and Woods' (1995) *Positive approaches to dementia care*. During this period in the UK, the Dementia Services Development Centres, pioneered by Professor

Mary Marshall, have been concerned with enhancing the psychosocial support provided to people with dementia, through training, education and consultancy for health and social care staff (Cantley 2005), with a similar centre in Norway (Engedal 2005). The Bradford Dementia Group, founded by Kitwood in 1992, is now an established academic Division of Dementia Studies at the University of Bradford, devoted to education and research in dementia.

The importance of subjectivity

Development within the person-centred approach contributed to and coincided with an interest in the subjectivity of people with dementia (e.g. Kitwood 1997b). Since the 1980s there have been a growing number of personal accounts of living with dementia (e.g. Harris 2002). The subjectivity of the experience is now considered not only worthy of exploration (Lyman 1989; Downs 1997) but essential to a full understanding and appropriate care provision, service development and evaluation (Cantley *et al.* 2005; Cotrell and Schulz 1993; Kitwood and Bredin 1992a, b). People with dementia are now becoming a political force in their own right organizing together in bodies such as the Dementia Advocacy Support Network International (www.dasninternational.org). In this way people with dementia are not only sharing their experience but in addition are maintaining and reclaiming their citizenship rights (Bartlett and O'Connor, 2007). The policy of user involvement in the UK (Department of Health 2001b) has yet to be fully implemented with people with dementia.

Person-centred care has promoted the value of looking at the world from the perspective of people with dementia, it has recognized the existence and importance of their life world, and their subjectivity. It has advocated for a bio-psychosocial approach to understanding dementia, incorporating biomedical understandings within a social context and personal life experiences. It has promoted understanding a person with dementia not only in terms of their own biography, but in the context of the wider net of social relationships of family and friends within which they are located. An emphasis on relationships and on communication also provides a creative environment in which to address the support needed by care staff.

Family members

An early concern with the use of the language of person-centred care was its apparent neglect, or even blame, of family members. Kitwood's (1997a) writings, however, do acknowledge the physical and emotional demands placed on family carers and stresses that unless family carers are well supported they will be unable to engage in person-centred care. Prior to the development of the person-centred approach to people with dementia there was recognition of the 'hidden victims' of dementia, the family carers (Zarit *et al.* 1985). (See Zarit, 2006 for a review of research on family carers). This led to an emphasis on service development designed to give carers a break (Jolley and Arie 1978) and, more recently, to an emphasis on the need for partnership working between professionals and family carers (Adams and Clarke 1999; Brodaty and Low 2005; Fortinsky 2001). For some, person-centred care places insufficient emphasis on those around the person with dementia, that is family members and care staff (Nolan *et al.* 2004). Nolan and colleagues prefer the term 'relationship-centred care' as it stresses the importance of addressing the needs of all of those affected by dementia (Nolan *et al.* 2004). They describe that it is not only people with dementia who have psychological needs but family and care staff also. These needs are captured in what Nolan *et al.* (2004) refer to as the senses framework. Woods and colleagues (2007) provide a useful guide for working with families, from this relationship-centred approach.

Changing the culture of care

The person-centred approach has come to be synonymous with practice development and organizational culture change. Kitwood and Benson (1995) wrote about the 'old' and 'new' culture of dementia care, arguing that person-centred care required that the needs of care staff and the organizational context within which much care for people with dementia is delivered deserved equal attention (Kitwood 1997a). We examine later, in Chapter 5, the extent to which there is a relationship between attempts to improve quality of care and improved quality of life for people with dementia. Kitwood and Bredin (1992) developed a methodology for assessing the extent to which a care setting was providing person-centred care. This they called Dementia Care Mapping (see Brooker 2005 for a review of this methodology). More recently Brooker (2007) proposed a framework for assessing the extent to which organizations practised person-centred care. This she refers to as the VIPS framework, where V refers to valuing people with dementia and those who work with them, I to the provision of individualized care, P to the need to adopt the perspective of a person with dementia, and S to the provision of a supportive social psychology.

Recent developments are addressing previously neglected areas of person-centred dementia care. For example, the broader sociopolitical context, while inferred, has not been explicitly addressed (Downs 2000; Innes 2002). This includes the effect of ethnicity and class on the experience of living with dementia (Bowes and Wilkinson 2003; Tibbs 2001). The physical environment of the buildings where people with dementia live and receive care is also known to influence people's experiences (Zeisel *et al.* 2003). Research and service development is being undertaken in these areas: for example Chalfont (2005) considers therapeutic design issues in long-term care settings for people with dementia. However, the potential of manipulating the care environment has yet to be fully incorporated into the person-centred model of care. Chalfont (2007) makes explicit the importance of access to nature and the role of the physical environment while Chaudhury (2002: 1999) describes how the environment can be used to support biography and life history. Calkins (2001) in the US and Marshall (2000) in the UK have been leading advocates of the therapeutic potential of the physical environment for people with dementia.

Until relatively recently, little explicit attention has been paid to the potential of the person-centred approach for people with dementia at the end of life. Hughes (2004) and Froggatt *et al.* (in press) have provided useful overviews linking both palliative and person-centred approaches. Hughes (2004) argues that at their core they both stress the inherent moral worth of the person, regardless of how ill or impaired they are. Elsewhere we have applied the key elements of the person-centred approach to those with severe dementia at the end of life, stressing that all of its principles and practices are as applicable to people at the end of life as they are to those earlier in the course of the condition (see Downs *et al.* 2006b). This includes an emphasis on communication and relationships, stimulation and engagement of the senses, physical care and comfort, spiritual care and attention to loss and grief.

As we have described, person-centred care is a term now frequently used in dementia care, although what it is used to describe differs. It may be that it is a term that is invoked rhetorically, and there is no guarantee that there is a shared value base between all those using the term. It is also present more generally in policy and service provision for older people. In the UK government's *National Service Framework for Older People* (Department of Health 2001a) there is an emphasis on treating people as individuals, a key tenet of person-centred care. This has led to a commitment to ensuring there are individualized packages of care. A challenge in this approach remains the need to consider the needs of the person and not prioritize addressing specific problems. That is, the point of any intervention should be on the whole context of a life – it should not be on any one symptom abstracted and isolated from its context (Brooker 2004). The tendency to consider isolated symptoms has also been reported in palliative care, despite one if its defining principles being a focus on the whole person (we examine this in more detail in Chapter 6).

What we have identified about care for people with dementia, in both clinical medicine and person-centred care, raises particular issues that may be more pronounced when we move to consider the needs of people with dementia at the end of life. Both old age psychiatry (Hughes 2004) and person-centred care (Downs *et al.* 2006b) are only recently turning their attention to care for people at the end of life. None of the approaches have given sustained attention to the place of dying and end of life issues. To allow us to engage with end of life care we will now consider the recent history for care for dying people before specifically examining care for people dying with dementia.

In summary, services for people with dementia have developed in response to a range of initiatives including those in clinical medicine and in person-centred care. These developments have been prompted and assisted by the advocacy efforts of family carers and, most recently, by people with dementia themselves. The last 30 years has seen an unprecedented growth in our understanding of the neurological, psychological and social aspects of living with dementia. We now turn our attention to similar developments in how we think about, and provide care to, those who are dying.

Care for people who are dying

In our consideration of the development of care for people who are dying, we focus on the origins of the hospice and palliative care movement and the guiding principles and practices that have been developed from it. We then consider the potential for this approach to end of life care for people with dementia.

The palliative care approach

In the years after the Second World War, first in the UK and subsequently in many parts of the world, a new way of responding to the care needs of people who were dying began to take shape. This new approach informed what became the modern hospice movement, palliative care and the pattern of bereavement care we now see in many countries. Pioneers began to shape a new paradigm that accepted the importance of embracing appropriate advances in medical science in the context of an ethical commitment to the importance of the self. Each individual should be supported to live as fully as possible until they died.

Four background factors contributed to shaping the development of hospices (Small 2000). First, the changing demographic and morbidity picture in the West. For example, by the beginning of the 1960s life expectancy in the UK had increased to 66.2 years for men and 71.2 for women, and has continued to increase since. Death from infectious disease had almost disappeared and most deaths were from circulatory or respiratory disease or from cancer (OPCS 1985). Secondly, treatments were developed that were relevant and effective for the typical client group of the hospices, that is people with advanced cancer. From the 1950s, clinical pharmacology and pain research were able to make considerable advances. Important articles on pain were published in the late 1950s and early 1960s (see summary in Clark 1998; Seymour *et al.* 2005) which led to the possibility of better pain management.

Thirdly, a growing body of research and anecdotal evidence that was critical of existing practice in the care of older people and of the dying. A series of studies identified the poor quality of care for older people and for people with cancer. Continued revelations, from the early 1950s until the 1980s, under-lined the intractability of the problem (Mellor and Shilling 1993). These studies included one which found many cancer patients, 'living on their own, or with equally old or infirm relatives, often in appalling housing conditions and often short of the right sort of food, warm clothing and bedding' (Marie Curie Memorial Foundation 1952: 18). Fourth, there was a shift in the way we understood death and bereavement in society. The range of critical scholar-ship about death and dying expanded in the post-war years (Mulkay and Ernst 1991; Corr 1993; Small 2000). Gorer (1955) described society as manifesting an increasing distance from death as a natural reality. Glaser and Strauss looked at 'awareness contexts' of the dying person (Glaser and Strauss 1965) and the differing trajectories of dying (Glaser and Strauss 1968), and at the idea that people left alone in hospital beds as they approached death first suffered a 'social death'. Shunned as a medical failure, Strauss and Glaser identify, in the case history of Mrs Abel, a 54-year-old woman dying of cancer, 'the lingering death of an increasingly isolated and rejected woman experiencing ever-growing pain'. Mrs Abel's last words before the operation from which she never recovered were, 'I hope I die' (Strauss and Glaser 1977: 21). Ariès (1974) identified five basic patterns in attitudes towards death in Western society from the middle ages to the present. He categorized the last of these as 'forbidden death' in which the subject is perceived as socially unacceptable, and is removed from social view, for example, into institutions, reflected in the experiences just described.

These background factors were necessary, but not sufficient, to effect the change that hospice and palliative care heralded in the way we care for the dying. The vision and tenacity of pioneers was the additional factor. This was inspired by an understanding of what was necessary, what was now possible, and a vision of what was desirable. By the early 1960s there were a few long-established hospices run by religious orders, in the UK, Ireland, the United States, and Australia. Cancer Care Inc. had been established in New York by social workers, the Marie Curie organization had ten homes in the UK and there were 19 beds for care of the terminally ill at the Royal Cancer Hospital (now the Royal Marsden Hospital) in London (Lamerton 1980). The birth of the modern hospice movement is widely linked with the opening of St Christopher's

Hospice in south London in 1967. The opening of St Christopher's was not the beginning of the story but only a significant milestone on the route (Clark 1998). Dame Cicely Saunders identified the origin of her ideas, that came to fruition in St Christopher's, in her clinical work during the 1940s.

Others were also contributing innovative work. In the USA Elizabeth Kübler-Ross, in 1969, published what became an international best-selling book, *On death and dying*, based on more than 500 interviews with dying patients (Kübler-Ross 1969). She subsequently summarized her thinking, both about society and institutional care, thus; 'We live in a very particular death-denying society. We isolate both the dying and the old, and it serves a purpose. They are reminders of our own mortality' (Kübler-Ross, evidence to US Senate Special Committee on Ageing 1972 – see www.nahc.org/HAA/history).

America's first hospice, The Connecticut Hospice Inc. in Branford, Connecticut, opened in 1974. Subsequently, there was a considerable emphasis on home care in the US. In Europe there was a significant early history of hospice care in both France and Ireland (Clark 2000). However, in terms of the modern hospice movement, it was the late 1970s, but particularly the 1980s, that saw significant growth. A home care service opened in Sweden in 1977 and in Italy in 1980. An inpatient unit started in Cologne, Germany in 1983, a palliative care unit in Santander, Spain, in 1984, a home care and inpatient unit in Belgium in 1985 and an inpatient hospice in the Netherlands in 1991 (Clark 2000).

The hospice pioneers recognized that medical science was making progress and that it was important to take advantage of all the tools in the modern pharmacoepia, but they also emphasized an idea of the importance of the self as something to be supported to live until death. The stance one adopted towards the dying was understood using the constructs of Christianity and understandings of the self drew on modern philosophies that were seeking to examine choice and responsibility, for example, those of Victor Frankl and Martin Buber.[2] At a 'Caring for Cancer' Conference in London (20 April 1998) Dame Cicely Saunders reminded people that the hospice movement, 'grew by listening' and embodied the basic philosophy that, 'You matter because you are you' and that people should be 'helped to live until they die' (Saunders 1998: 6–7).

---

[2] We have identified Buber as an influence on person-centred dementia care. We will further explore the way Buber's work has been looked to and developed in subsequent chapters.

As with person-centred dementia care described earlier, enthusiasts for hospice and palliative care would have it identified as 'a philosophy not a facility' (Corr and Corr 1983). 'The central point about hospice is the outlook, attitude, or approach it represents, not the building or structure in which it may be housed' (Corr *et al.* 2004: 227). Hospice is best understood then not as a noun but 'as an adjective that is best used in two ways: (1) to single out a particular philosophy of care, and (2) to identify the organized programmes that seek to implement or deliver that care' (Corr *et al.* 2004: 227). If we accept this, the hospice influences can be identified in a wide range of activity, from palliative care (Box 3.3) and bereavement care to a propagation of multiprofessional working and a holistic approach to responding to need.

Box 3.3 Definition of palliative care

Palliative care is an approach that improves the quality of life of patients and their families facing the problem associated with life-threatening illness, through the prevention and relief of suffering by means of early identification and impeccable assessment and treatment of pain and other problems, physical, psychosocial and spiritual.

Palliative care:

- provides relief from pain and other distressing symptoms;
- affirms life and regards dying as a normal process;
- intends neither to hasten or postpone death;
- integrates the psychological and spiritual aspects of patient care;
- offers a support system to help patients live as actively as possible until death;
- offers a support system to help the family cope during the patients' illness and in their own bereavement;
- uses a team approach to address the needs of patients and their families, including bereavement counselling, if indicated;
- will enhance quality of life, and may also positively influence the course of illness;
- is applicable early in the course of illness, in conjunction with other therapies that are intended to prolong life, such as chemotherapy or radiation therapy, and includes those investigations needed to better understand and manage distressing clinical complications.

(World Health Organization 2002)

Current service provision for people who are dying is present in mainstream services in the UK (Box 3.4) and worldwide (Box 3.5)

Whilst the provision described in Boxes 3.4 and 3.5 is largely for people with cancer, the spread and impact of hospices goes wider. The diversification of hospice and specialist palliative care services continues today in different ways relevant to the disease people die with, their stage in the life cycle and the types of services that a country can offer. Other settings of care that are receiving

Box 3.4 Figures for UK hospice and palliative care services – 2005

Inpatient units:

220 for adults (29 per cent NHS managed) – 3156 beds (33 units with 255 beds)

Adult patient statistics for 2003–4:

- ◆ Inpatient admissions a year 58,000
- ◆ Estimated number of deaths in palliative care units 30,000
- ◆ Mean length of stay in hospice 13 days
- ◆ 95 per cent of patients had cancer
- ◆ 32 per cent under 65 years old (9 per cent over 84)
- ◆ Estimated 18 per cent of cancer deaths occurring in palliative care units

Community and hospital support services – 2005

- ◆ 358 Home care services
- ◆ 104 Hospice at Home services
- ◆ 263 Day care services
- ◆ 68 Hospital support nurses
- ◆ 293 Hospital support teams

Adult patient statistics for 2004–5:

- ◆ 155 000 patients seen by community services
- ◆ Estimated number of deaths at home 38,000
- ◆ 70 per cent of cancer deaths cared for by home care teams
- ◆ 32,000 patients cared for annually in day care (excludes Scotland)

(Hospice Information Service 2006)

Box 3.5 Worldwide figures

- ◆ 50 million deaths a year
- ◆ 3.1 million died of AIDS in 2004 (39.4 million have HIV/AIDS)
- ◆ 6 million cancer deaths a year
- ◆ Estimated 15 million new cases of cancer every year by 2020 (www.who.int – see also www.unaids.org)
- ◆ Hospice and palliative care projects in approx 100 countries, over 8,000 initiatives
- ◆ USA 3,139 hospice and palliative care services
- ◆ Canada 650
- ◆ Australia 280
- ◆ France 91 inpatient units, 291 hospital-based palliative care teams

(Hospice Information Service 2006)

For other countries see the International Observatory on End-of Life Care at www.eolc-observatory.net.

increased attention as relevant to palliative care include community hospitals (Payne *et al.* 2004) and long-term care settings for older people (Froggatt 2004). There is also the provision of palliative care to people with conditions other than cancer (Addington-Hall 1998). Services for people with conditions other than cancer were initially for people with neurological conditions and HIV/AIDS, but now there is more attention paid to the needs of people with circulatory disorders (heart and lung failure), stroke, and also dementia (National Council for Palliative Care 2006). Children (American Academy of Pediatrics 2000) and older people (Davies and Higginson 2004) have also been singled out as groups in the population that may have different needs and requirements for palliative care.

The palliative care approach: consequences for people with dementia

The case for making palliative care available for people with dementia has been made on the grounds of equity, need and on the basis that adopting a palliative care approach would improve the quality of care available. These are the grounds used for all conditions when it is argued that palliative care should be made available for them (Addington-Hall 1998; Field and Addington-Hall 1999).

Further, it is likely that a considerable number of people have complex illness experiences, for example it is argued in the UK that approximately 9 per cent of people aged 75–84 years, and 29 per cent of people over 85 years, who die due to cancer, circulatory and respiratory conditions also have dementia (National Council for Palliative Care 2006). Symptom burden is similar in people with cancer compared to those with dementia (McCarthy *et al.* 1997: Mitchell *et al.* 2004) although the types of symptoms are likely to vary (Olsen 2003).

A quality argument is also used to make the case for service provision. A case is made that quality of care is poor for people with dementia, which leads to a poor quality of life and ultimately a poor dying. Palliative care is perceived to be the way in which to improve care, enhance a person with dementia's quality of life and ease their death. We will argue in Chapter 6 that the basis on which quality of care is identified is flawed, not least because it neglects the subjective world of the person, and we will argue that it is problematic to equate quality of care automatically with quality of life. Despite this the argument that palliative care has much to offer people with dementia is one that we support, and will develop.

There is little evidence that people with dementia are accessing mainstream palliative care services, although there are national variations. In the USA, admission of people with dementia into hospice programmes has been promoted since the early 1980s (Volicer 1986). In the UK, specialist palliative care teams and hospices are under-used by older people and by people with non-cancer diagnoses, including dementia (Lloyd-Williams 1996; Addington-Hall and Higginson 2001). In general, palliative care has had difficulties when prognosis is uncertain and when dying is potentially protracted (Hanrahan and Luchins 1995). Palliative care units have often not known how to respond to cognitive and behavioural problems (Luchins and Hanrahan 1993; Volicer *et al.* 1994; de Vries *et al.* in press). It is a situation in which the eminent head of a French regional palliative care service was able to say, in a plenary at a European conference, that; 'as a rule, patients suffering from dementia and wanting to be managed by a palliative care unit ought to remember to develop some form of cancer' (Wary 2003: 29).

A number of barriers to people with dementia accessing hospice and specialist palliative care have been identified (Hancock *et al.* 2006; Robinson *et al.* 2005a). These barriers include a lack of recognition of dementia as a terminal illness, problems with prognostication, a deficit of skills and knowledge with respect to providing palliative care for people with dementia amongst care providers, including challenges in responding to behavioural aspects and communication with people with dementia. In the UK, the palliative care literature recognized that 'diseases manifesting a dementia syndrome are terminal illnesses' (Black and Jolley 1990: 1321) as early as 1990 but even 10 years later did not consider dementia as falling within their remit.

The challenges of prognostication for people with dementia can often be the key limitation to accessing specialist services. Hospice and specialist palliative care services characteristically provide time-limited interventions. As it is more difficult to predict how long a person with dementia might live, people with dementia may be denied access to these services. This is particularly pertinent in those countries, including the US, where funding for care, and specifically for hospice care, is limited to the last six weeks of life.

There is also a recognized deficit in skills and knowledge with respect to palliative care for people with dementia amongst care providers, in general, acute and primary care settings as well as in more specialist palliative care contexts. There is a need to acquaint palliative care staff with the progress that has been made in identifying the range and changing nature of needs that people with dementia will have. Death can occur at any time from age-associated conditions such as atrial fibrillation, heart failure and myocardial infarction. With increased immobility, weakness and swallowing difficulties the likely presence of a life-threatening physical illness increases (Burns *et al.* 1990; Jolley and Baxter 1997). Specifically, palliative care staff may find the challenges in communication with people with dementia a deterrent to providing care. Established practices in palliative care have been based on the person being cared for being able to articulate their needs and then inform staff if they have been met or not.

Another barrier is a concern that staff (and volunteers and financial supporters) would perceive dementia care as less rewarding (National Council for Hospice and Specialist Palliative Care Services and Scottish Partnership Agency for Palliative and Cancer Care 2000). This also has implications for the future funding of services in the UK. Charitable giving underpins much of the funding for hospices and it is feared by some within hospices that the alleviation of the suffering of dementia in older adults is not such an attractive cause to take to potential financial donors compared to the needs of younger people dying with cancer. One should not assume, however, that social attitudes will remain the same. An increase in the number of older people in all Western societies and an anticipated corresponding increase in the number of people living with dementia may change the public perceptions about the worthiness of this area. Further, as cancer treatments develop and people live longer after a cancer diagnosis they may also develop dementia.

Care for people with dementia who are dying

We have identified that a case can be made for the provision of palliative care for people with dementia. Despite the presence of recognized barriers to the development and provision of such services, there are pockets of small-scale service provision that exist, usually linked to pioneering individuals.

In considering palliative care services for people with dementia, it is necessary to recognize that palliative care can be provided in three ways (National Council for Hospices and Specialist Palliative Care Services 1995):

1. Specialist palliative care – done in and by units with palliative care as their core specialty, with accredited staff. Found in inpatient units, hospital palliative care teams, day care, specialist community services, hospices.

2. General palliative care – should be used by every doctor or nurse caring for a person nearing the end of a chronic illness, it is an integral part of all clinical practice. Applicable everywhere – at home, through general practice, hospitals, nursing and residential homes.

3. Palliative procedures and techniques – mostly performed by specialists in other disciplines e.g. radiotherapy, chemotherapy, psychosocial care.

The services that do exist for people with dementia range from specialist units specifically for people with severe dementia through to the promotion of a palliative care approach, or general palliative care, to be provided wherever the person with dementia resides. This latter approach is one advocated in recent UK government policy in the White Paper, 'Your health, your care, your say' (Department of Health 2006a) which included an intention to seek to improve care for people dying in any setting with any condition.

Whilst the current evidence of the impact of initiatives that promote a palliative care approach in advanced dementia in hospitals is limited (Sampson *et al.* 2005), there are an increasing number of descriptive accounts that we will now summarize.

Specialist palliative care units for people with dementia

The first specialist palliative care services for people with dementia were developed in the United States. Subsequently, there have been new initiatives in Europe and Australia. These services take on one of two forms: programmes of palliative care delivered in established care settings (Volicer *et al.* 1994; Ahronheim *et al.* 2000; Abbey *et al.* 2006), or a stand-alone hospice unit in a long-term care facility (Wilson *et al.* 1996; Kovach 1997). The development of palliative care provision as a part of the activity of established teams and settings has seen activity in people's homes (Hanrahan and Luchins 1995; Shega *et al.* 2003; Treolar 2006), in hospitals (Abbey *et al.* 2006; Ahronheim *et al.* 2000) and in long-term care settings (Volicer *et al.* 1994). For example, Kovach (1997) describes a late-stage dementia care programme which is based on palliative care principles in Box 3.6. With its origins in the dementia care world, this contrasts with less focused programmes developed by hospices in the US which provide support for people with dementia in whatever setting the person resides (Corr *et al.* 2004; Brechling and Kuhn 1989; Brenner 1998).

In Australia, research is being undertaken to establish a model of multidisciplinary palliative care for people with end-stage dementia living in residential aged care facilities incorporating case conferences (Abbey *et al.* 2006). The development and piloting of this model of multidisciplinary palliative care has recently been completed and indicates that further work is required. The case conference provided an opportunity for all interested parties to share information about the residents' conditions and wishes regarding care at the end of life.

Box 3.6 Late-stage dementia care program philosophy

The late-stage dementia household is a home for residents with late-stage Alzheimer's disease and other dementing illnesses. The household provides a nurturing, safe, and stimulating environment with an emphasis on maintaining personhood, comfort, quality of life, and human dignity. Holistic needs of the residents are met through an interdisciplinary therapeutic approach to care. The household is committed to meeting the needs of the resident–family dyad.

Goals:

- To provide a home for people with late-stage dementia that is safe, therapeutic, dignified, and life-affirming and that provides a sense of security
- To provide therapies and programs that provide comfort, personhood, quality of life, and human dignity
- To balance inner retreat activities with socially connected activities so that residents do not become overwhelmed or overburdened
- To allow residents to set their own pace and style of participation, whether that is initiating, observing, or actively participating
- To prevent physical iatrogenic (caused by the treatment or setting) problems
- To maintain, nurture, and value a sense of family ties and positive family involvement
- To provide the resources and atmosphere needed for staff to be able to actualize the philosophy and goals of the program and to give and receive support from one another

(Kovach 1997)

Whilst the aim is to ensure the provision of comfort care, some of these services aim to go beyond just physical care to address issues of personhood and meaning, as illustrated in Kovach's 1997 programme in Box 3.6.

With one exception (Shega *et al.* 2003) all these programmes are provided for people with dementia who are identified as having advanced or end-stage dementia. They are often bed-bound and require total physical care and support (e.g. Abbey *et al.* 2006; Kovach 1997; Hanrahan and Luchins 1995; Hanrahan *et al.* 1999). The exception is Shega *et al.* (2003) who have established, in the United States, a liaison team based in primary geriatric practice. This aims to support people with dementia much earlier in their illness through to their death, with an emphasis on end of life care.

Development of general palliative care for people with dementia

Current provision of care for people with dementia at the end of life in general care settings is not always appropriate, as illustrated in Chapter 2, despite the level of need being high. A recent retrospective case note audit of an acute

Box 3.7 Model of multidisciplinary palliative care for residents with end-stage dementia

Setting: two residential aged care facilities (RACF)

Elements of model:

♦ RACF staff education about palliative care

♦ Multidisciplinary care conference using enhanced primary care guidelines and implementation of palliative goals

♦ Liaison between palliative care service, residents, relatives, RACF staff and General Practitioner also available.

Process:

Model piloted for 10 months with 17 residents

Outcomes:

♦ Twelve case conferences conducted

♦ Nutrition and hydration discussed in case conferences

♦ Family satisfaction with care high following a case conference

♦ Further refinement and evaluation required

(Abbey *et al.* 2006)

medical ward in a London hospital in the UK indicated that one in four older adults dying on the ward had dementia (Sampson *et al.* 2006). The overall experience of people dying with dementia in hospitals, as has been shown, is characterized by more invasive treatments than a comparable group of people with a cancer diagnosis (Ahronheim *et al.* 1996). Further, they are less likely to receive palliative care interventions than people without a dementia diagnosis (Sampson *et al.* 2006). A similar pattern of care has also been identified in the home setting in Japan (Hirakawa 2006).

The development of general palliative care for people with dementia in settings such as hospitals and long-term care settings is supported in two ways. There are care setting-specific initiatives. These are designed to improve the care of all people dying in any particular setting, for example long-term care facilities, or hospitals. There are also a range of initiatives being promoted to help prepare generalist care practitioners for meeting the needs of people living and dying with dementia.

Site-specific initiatives that have relevance for people dying with dementia are largely seen in the area of long-term care. In many Western countries much effort has been directed at improving the provision of palliative care (see for example Australian Government Department of Health and Ageing 2004, Froggatt 2004, Parker-Oliver *et al.* 2004). Specific work to promote palliative care for people with dementia has utilized guidelines (Lloyd-Williams and Payne 2002), and the provision of educational programmes (Kovach 1997; Abbey *et al.* 2006). These guidelines may be linked to specific care settings, for example, residential aged care facilities in Australia, (Australian Government Department of Health and Ageing 2004), or long-stay hospital settings in the UK (Lloyd-Williams and Payne 2002).

Some guidelines focus on practical care issues such as the management of pain and the use of syringe drivers for pain management, vomiting, agitation, oral care, constipation, breathlessness, fevers, and pressure care (Lloyd-Williams and Payne 2002). Others offer a broader perspective including the principles of palliation, issues of dignity, advance care planning, assessment and management of physical symptoms, psychological, social, spiritual, and family support (Australian Government Department of Health and Ageing 2004).

We can also identify, in initiatives established to develop certain aspects of dementia care, congruence with palliative care provision. For example, The Good Sunset Project in Australia (Box 3.8) included a specific focus on end-of-life care through staff development work and The Good Sunset Project.

Box 3.8 The Good Sunset Project (Killick and Allan 2006)

Aim: To better communicate with people with dementia, to understand people's experiences and needs and to improve their quality of life

Project design – three elements:

1. Staff initiatives – four communication projects
2. Getting Through Initiative based on coma care work principles with 4 residents with advanced dementia
3. End of Life Group – regular meetings with managers

Outcomes of getting through initiative:

- Genuine communication identified with three residents
- Questions raised about what this communication meant
- Time-intensive work
- Closure of communication work difficult
- No longer-term evaluation of benefits for individuals

Downloaded from www.hammond.com.au/dsdc/projects.php, 26 November 2006

Specific interventions Many interventions could be deemed palliative and supportive for people with dementia as they encompass all aspects of clinical care. It is not the intention of this book to provide information about how to meet specific clinical needs of individuals with dementia, as an increasing number of texts are available which provide just such information (See de Vries 2003; Hughes 2005; Miesen and Jones 2006). Characteristically, within the texts, the focus is on one clearly defined individual symptom at a time. Ways to identity and meet specific problems through the delivery of specific interventions are suggested. This breakdown into small elements and numerous foci is understandable, but the challenge is how to integrate such elements to provide all-encompassing care.

Another example of a palliative intervention for a person with dementia towards the end of life focuses on improving communication. The Good Sunset Project (Box 3.8), mentioned above, is one such example. It utilizes the principles of coma care for people with dementia (Barnes and Tomandl 2004). Coma care work is an approach developed for people in comas to facilitate ways of communication in situations where communication seemed to be impossible, or very difficult. An underlying value is that whilst a person is breathing, there is consciousness and love and connection can still be imparted and made (Tomandl 1991). The principles of coma care work are in-depth communication, communication from cues, the use of multiple channels of communication including sight, hearing, sound, body sensation, and touch, and the seeking of positive feedback from the person. The consequences of such an approach for the person with dementia and for their relative are described in Box 3.9.

This emphasis on strategies to enhance communication between the person with dementia and another person is consistent with both the principles of person-centred care and palliative care, but it relies on identifying strategies from other areas of health care and translating them for use to meet the specific needs of a person with dementia.

Box 3.9 An experience of coma care

Rosemary Clarke describes how she has used coma care work to communicate with her 91-year-old mother, who has dementia and has lived with this for six years at the time of her writing.

This is how my mother and I between us interpreted coma work to our benefit.

On arriving in my mother's room, I settled myself very close beside her in such a way that I could speak into her ear and at the same time have my finger-tips on her wrist, at least to start with. Usually this entailed me kneeling to one side of her reclining chair or her bed. There was typically no response from her at this stage, though very occasionally she turned to me. Next, I checked carefully what activity my mother was already engaged in. Typically she would, for example, be looking or chewing (she did that a lot), or moving one finger a tiny bit. She might even be moving her facial muscles or even a foot. She might sigh. Any event was important.

I would then focus on one of these, the most energetic or striking, to begin with. With my voice and sometimes also with my hand (or just a finger) I would support my mother to 'go with' that little impulse, to give it its fullest expression. Always I was following her lead, never suggesting or initiating.

Almost all of the meetings we had were spent with my index finger and her thumb in a constant 'dance': pressure from her thumb was replied to with the same pressure from my finger at the same speed. Sometimes the dance was slow and soft, at other times I was firm, insistent, at other times very pressing.

(Clarke 2004: 23)

While it is possible to identify examples of innovative practice there remain challenges in disseminating lessons learned more widely. There are also particular groups of people who have dementia, who appear to be less well served. These include younger people with dementia (Keady and Nolan 1994) and people from ethnic minorities (Bowes and Wilkinson 2003). People in these groups occupy the margins within the margins.

As we discussed above, there is also a dimension to palliative care that is best captured as a particular approach to the relationship between self, illness and society. We will conclude this section by looking at one area that has developed alongside hospice and palliative care, that of the understanding of bereavement and loss. We will consider the ways the insights of this new understanding can link with dementia care.

Bereavement and loss

Developments in hospice and palliative care drew on emerging debates about understanding death in society and about the meaning of care and the importance of the self. We have also argued that many of these debates have resonance for understanding the individual impact and social significance of dementia and for shaping service provision. We will use the example of developing conceptualization of the bereavement process and the potential for bereavement care to illustrate the links that can be made between aspects of palliative care and dementia care.

Those links are made easier to elaborate because of the coincidence of shared origins via the work of John Bowlby. Bereavement care in the modern hospice movement was shaped by an early encounter in London between Cicely Saunders and Colin Murray Parkes (Clark *et al.* 2005: 159–60). Dr Parkes was working with John Bowlby, who is described in the dedication in Volume 1 of *Care giving in dementia* as the person 'who unknowingly provided the concept of attachment history which turned out to be a fundamental key to be able to relate to the inner world of the demented elderly' (Jones and Miesen 1992).

A number of landmark developments in thinking about bereavement can be used to help understand the challenges of dementia care and the impact of progressive dementia. Glaser and Strauss (1965) spoke of the emotional awareness of terminally ill patients about their condition. This emotional awareness may also be evident in people with dementia. Miesen argues that 'even demented persons experience and feel threatened losses' (Miesen 1992: 39).

Rando, originally in 1986 and then in a more refined form in 2000, developed her understanding of anticipatory grief/anticipatory mourning (Rando 1986, 2000). She portrayed mourning as a reaction to all losses encountered in the past, present or in the future of a life-threatening illness. This describes the everyday reality for many people with dementia and for people caring for someone with dementia, as they watch successive losses and anticipate those losses to come (Doka 2004: 2).

A paper by Kalish (1966) presented the concept of 'psychological death' – a loss of individual consciousness in which a person ceases to be aware of self. 'Not only does he not know who he is – he does not know that he is' (Kalish 1966: 247). It is an experience that resonates with Ignatieff's fictional narrator talking about his mother who has dementia in his novel *Scar Tissue*. Here he is discussing the likely future with his mother's doctor. The doctor tells him:

> 'Her semantic and syntactic memory functions have collapsed, but prosodic variation is still intact' Prosodic variation means tone of voice, facial expression, gestures – some patients drawl or stutter in a voice they have never heard before. 'They hear themselves speak and they think who is this'. It is the word 'still' that bothers me.
>
> (Ignatieff 1993: 58)

Later in the novel, after further deterioration in his mother he describes a point of crisis: 'I had arrived at the moment, long foretold, hopelessly prepared for, when Mother took the step beyond her self and moved into the world of death with her eyes open' (Ignatieff 1993: 166).

Doka and Aber (2002), in relation to dementia, consider how family members experience 'the death of the person who once was'. Spouses, they argue, may become 'crypto widows'. (This consideration of psychological death is problematic given the arguments we have presented about prevailing assumptions as to the nature of the self.) Linda Grant's book *Remind me who I am, again* (1998) is about the diagnosis of multi-infarct dementia in her mother, Rose Grant, in 1993, and her mother's subsequent need for care both from her daughters and from social services and care homes. She deals with the difficult issues of deciding that she wants her mother to be cared for in a care home and addresses the question about the nature of the self in the context of all the changes in her mother. The head of the care home says to Linda:

> How do you relate to people when you are re-inventing yourself and the situation almost as you go along? That's what your mother does. How else could she do it? In a way your mother is dead and in a way she's not dead. But you're equally dead because you're not the child she carried through to whatever point. So how do you hang on to whatever sense you have of who that person really was, is and should be about, so that you don't just stick them in a box somewhere and forget about it and at the same time recognize the reality that you have to let go.
>
> (Grant 1998: 268)

Doka (1989) has argued for the importance of recognizing the existence of 'disenfranchised grief'. This refers to an idea that certain people are not identified as legitimate grievers after a death (it is an idea that draws on the experience of gay men being excluded from the funeral arrangements made for their partner by their partner's biological family. But it also evident in an expectation that professionals and even family in some cases are not expected to feel grief and hence are not offered any support.) There is a culturally prevalent belief that the death of a person with dementia is a release, for carer and for the person with dementia – that they are old and a 'burden' and that death must be 'welcomed'. In relation to staff grief, unlike hospices where a person may only have been an inpatient for a short period of time before their death, long-term care staff may have known a person with dementia for some years. Katz *et al.* (2000) identified the need for bereavement support for the staff involved in long-term care relationships.

The debate that is most prominent in bereavement scholarship in recent years is one that contrasts an idea that one must 'move on' from loss, establishing a new identify shaped without continuing reference to the person who has died, and an approach that affirms the importance of 'continuing bonds' – the dead continuing in an ongoing role in the lives of the living (see Klass *et al.* 1996, Walter 1996, Small 2001). The significance for the losses associated with the progression of dementia is that the continuing bonds approach suggests one can engage with the person that *was* while not denying the challenges of living with the person that *is*.[3]

The example of responses to bereavement gives an insight into the rich potential for combining palliative care, geriatric medicine and dementia care. Combining approaches could benefit pain and symptom control at the end of life, it could enhance psychological and social care. Combined approaches would involve work with whole family helping them celebrate life that is left to live and reconcile to the loss of capacities and to future bereavement. It would also engage with the negative attitudes of society through arguing that the self was retained and that positive things could be achieved for people with dementia and for their families and communities.

The system world in context

From these accounts of the history of dementia care and hospice and palliative care we can identify several common threads that have a place in the system world. These include:

1. The segregation from mainstream services of older people, people with dementia and people who are dying;

---

[3] We have presented this argument in Small *et al.* 2006: 379–81.

2. The importance of innovation that has developed in response to perceived deficits in care and, concurrently, through innovative examples of good practice often led by the insights of practitioners and patients;

3. The recognition of the need to go beyond one approach, or the contribution of one discipline, to develop multidisciplinary and multifaceted working;

4. A recognition that one should address all of a person's needs, that is one should not consider a particular need in isolation; and

5. The privileging of the subjective experience of the person living with the condition in the construction of a new ethic of care (Small *et al.* 2006).

These new assumptions about the way one should care for people with dementia are challenging, not least because they cross that boundary between the life-world and system world. The life-world should shape the services that are offered, as opposed to the system world deciding what individuals need. Services shaped by life-world concerns are likely to mean that, for example, while it is necessary to achieve as full a control of a person's physical needs as possible, if this is achieved it is not the end of treatment. One can then move on to address their social, psychological and spiritual needs.

Conclusions

In this chapter we have examined the discourses that have underpinned service development in dementia care and care for dying people. In particular we have concentrated on clinical medicine and person-centred care. We have looked at care for people with dementia and care for people who are dying and have considered how far each can support the other. There has been a continuing development of the possibilities offered by clinical medicine, but there are also developments that are based on the centrality of respecting and supporting the self. There is also much critical thinking about the nature of dementia and its relationship with society, including an engagement with the ethics of care.

We have considered the current provision of services for people with dementia, with a specific focus on what is provided when they are deemed to be dying. We can conclude that for people journeying with dementia, there are some services designed to meet their needs with respect to their dying. In general they are not made available until they are near death. Services that do exist are limited in number, fragmented, and largely focused on the physiological and functional aspects of living with advanced dementia and they are largely institutionally based. The possibilities to consider one's dying are rarely made available at diagnosis or early in the dementia journey.

We need to consider the psychological, social and spiritual needs of individuals during the entire journey with dementia, and the diversity of needs that arise for people whose age and ethnicity takes them outside the majority groupings for people with dementia (these majority groupings are 'old' and 'white'). Whilst person-centred care creates a space for subjective experience the attention to diversity in this experience has yet to be fully developed.

The discourses of clinical medicine, person-centred care and palliative care have helped us to understand why people's journeys are sometimes at odds with the service worldview of the disease and its presentation of needs and problems. A limitation of much of what we have described has been an implicit assumption that dementia is a discrete condition and this is the only focus of care and support. The reality for many people, as we described in Chapter 2, is that dementia is but one of several conditions a person may be living with and the presence of dementia may either mask other conditions, or it may itself be ignored.

Much of the dissonance we see in terms of care and support services provided for people with dementia and their families reflects underlying ambivalences held by wider society to ageing, dying and dementia. Dementia, and people associated with it (people with dementia, their family members, care staff) find themselves in an ambiguous position with respect to society. Whilst calls are made for it to be recognized as a terminal condition, this is not reflected in how services and support are provided, where the greater emphasis is on living. Ignoring dying prevents attention being paid to appropriate management of this final part of a person's life.

We go on to examine these issues further in the following chapters by focusing on:

◆ a consideration of constructions of self and identity for the individual

◆ what underpins service drivers in the system world

◆ the way in which the dying and death are conceptualized and managed.

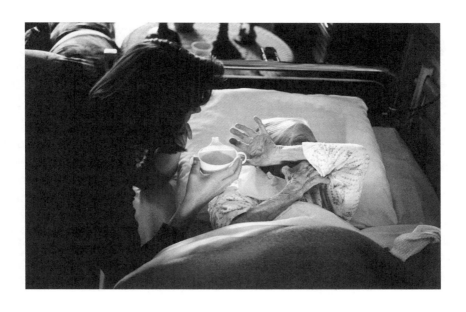

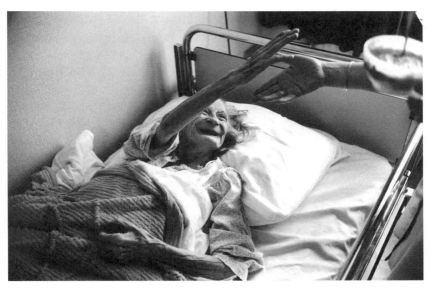

Chapter 4

Self and autonomy

I've been towing the content of my origins but the
ground is very uneven, but I'm leaving literature in the
thin patches.
Alan Kidd

Troubling autonomy

The concept of individuals having choices about the provision of their health
and social care is deemed to be a key value across the British public sector.
This emphasis on choice can be identified in policies related to both palliative
care and care for older people (Froggatt 2005). A key component of the prevailing construct of choice is a focus on individual autonomy. If we are to
understand why it is that people with dementia receive the care they do we
need to examine whether an approach based on autonomy is the most appropriate basis for ensuring quality of care in dementia. The construct of an
autonomous individual is only one way of approaching an understanding of
what constitutes the self. In this chapter we will present an argument in favour
of a relational view of self in dementia. We will argue that people with dementia will be best served by recognizing our essential interdependence and con-
nectivity. We will propose that an emphasis on individual autonomy not only
excludes people with dementia but undermines the potential of communities
to be a focus for care.

Considering the nature of the self in people with dementia brings life-world
and system worlds into conflict. As we have seen in the previous chapter, some
of the influential world views of dementia seen within clinical medicine are
primarily concerned with assessing and treating a person's experience in terms
of objective and measurable signs and symptoms. From such a perspective, much
of what a person with dementia experiences and expresses is seen as a manifestation of their symptomatology. The life-world view as told through narrative,
literature and the arts, on the other hand, suggests that much of what the person

experiences is understandable as a search for, and a construction of, meaning. Further, much of the meaning made has internal consistency and connects with the actions they undertake.

Interest in what constitutes self and in the interaction of self and the system world requires us to engage with postmodern considerations about different forms of reason: scientific; moral/practical; and aesthetic. We introduced these differences in Chapter 1. From the perspective of scientific reason, with its focus on objectivity, cognition is a prerequisite for self and if cognition is disrupted by dementia, then dementia leads to disruption or loss of self. From a moral practical approach to reason, self is present in people with dementia but requires the cooperation of others to be upheld and affirmed (Kitwood 1994). While from an aesthetic perspective on reason, even if self is diminished the mere act of being entitles one to moral personhood (Jennings 2000; Post 2000ab).

In this chapter, we will challenge the widespread assumption that self is inevitably destroyed by dementia and propose that, while self may be changed, it can be preserved. We will demonstrate that to assume intact cognition is a requirement for the existence of self limits our imagination when it comes to our relationship with people with dementia. Most importantly, we will question whether autonomy should be the guiding principle in the care for people with dementia.

Concern with the nature of the self in people with dementia is not just an academic exercise. How we conceptualize the key characteristics of what it means to have a self, and any changes brought to it by dementia, will affect our response to people with dementia. A view that dementia destroys the self and thus the very essence of what it means to be human is widespread, but it is not the only view. Both within philosophical and practice circles argument and evidence have been marshalled in support of the view that the self is not completely eroded when living with dementia. While such arguments recognize that the self and its expression may be changed, they argue that self is more than cognition. In this chapter we locate these views within different philosophical traditions and include narratives from people with dementia and family members that explore this argument.

Broadly speaking, self can be regarded as being cognitive or relational. In this chapter we argue that self is not constituted solely in terms of cognition but is inhibited and facilitated by the behaviour and practices of others, be they health and social care professionals, family members or people in local neighbourhoods. This relational view of self leads to different ways of viewing and engaging with the person with dementia, including different ways of thinking about autonomy. It leads us towards a different ethic of care.

A cognitively constituted self

If human beings are constituted by cognition, memory and reasoning, the very faculties which are affected by brain disease, then dementia leads to loss of self. The idea that dementia 'destroys the selfhood of its victims' is widespread (Ballenger 2006: 152, see also Herskovits 1995) and lies at the heart of our concern with dementia as the dread disease of contemporary times. Perhaps it is not surprising that dementia has been associated with loss of self given the close links we make between mind and self. The term dementia is based on the Latin *demens*, meaning mad, and the French word *dement*, without mind. Berrios (2000) describes the link between dementia and impaired reasoning being made as early as the eighteenth century.

The English empiricist philosopher John Locke (1632–1704) argued that what makes a person a person is self-consciousness, the capacity to think and to reflect on their own existence. In contemporary terms we would call this reflexivity. This view provides a theoretical and philosophical basis for the argument that someone with dementia who has no personal memories, while biologically alive, has no self.

In contemporary times Parfit (1984) comes closest to representing this Lockean view. According to Mathews (2006), for Parfit, self requires cognitive functioning such as reason and memory. It is reason and memory that allows a person to retain a continuous 'I' despite changes in their life. To be oneself requires 'psychological continuity' whereby one thinks of oneself as oneself, by continuing to remember one's past. If I no longer remember my past life I lack 'psychological continuity'. I am no longer the person I was. From this perspective, people with progressive cognitive impairment experience a gradual deterioration of personhood or self. They lack the requisite 'inner goings on' that, for Parfit, are essential to having self.

Loss of self is then equated with 'death' in a hybrid construction such as in the tile of Woods' (1989) book, *Alzheimer's disease: Coping with a living death*. This theme is also present in Cohen and Eisdorfer's (1986) book *The Loss of Self*, where they describe two kinds of death (1986: 259): (1) physical death; and (2) psychological death or 'the death of the self' which, they argue, precedes physical death by many years.

> the ongoing psychological death of the patient causes profound grief, and the grieving is very much like the reaction to terminal illness, but with one major difference. The patient appears healthy, looks very much like he or she used to look, and is likely to be alive for many months or years in this peculiar state of physical health and psychological decline. It is not easy to deal with the invisible changes that alter behaviour and mood and destroy the husband, wife, patient, or friend whom one has known for years … Although we may actually do more for the patient as he or she becomes more

dependent, we also begin to regard the patient as the shell of someone we once knew – much as we treasure an object we inherited for its power to evoke memories of another time. It is hard to say that this distancing process is wrong. The greatest danger of distancing is that the patient becomes an object – a flesh and blood container holding memories and deep emotional ties to the past but with no real function of humanity in the present.

(Cohen and Eisdorfer 1986: 260–1)

Words like 'a shell', 'an object', and of 'having no function' all represent aspects of this living death, which are also described here in the diary of someone with dementia:

> No theory of medicine can explain what is happening to me. Every few months I sense that another piece of me is missing. My life ... my self ... are falling apart. I can only think half thoughts now. Someday I may wake up and not think at all ... not know who I am. Most people expect to die someday, but who ever expected to lose their self first.

(Cohen and Eisdorfer 1986: 22)

This idea that selfhood is destroyed in dementia has been used in media campaigns by advocacy groups including the Alzheimer's Society in the UK and the US Alzheimer's Association. Bender *et al.* (2002) cite research on determinants of successful fund-raising campaigns for intellectual disability charities which suggest that donations are greatest when they prompt guilt about, and sympathy for, the person rather than when they present the person as being capable, having value and having rights. They asked 38 people to rank ten posters used for fund-raising purposes by the Alzheimer's Society in the UK. They note that while such posters are good for charities in terms of income generation, they succeed at the price of serving to support the negative stereotyping and negative social role valuation of people with dementia.

The perceived effect of cognition on self is illustrated below by an interview on BBC Radio Four on 8 November 2005. At the beginning of the programme David Whitcombe, a person with dementia, introduces himself in the following way: 'I'm David Whitcombe and I've got Alzheimer's disease.'

Later in the radio broadcast, after discussing the effect dementia has had upon him, he refers to himself as now being *David Witless*. With reference to his wife he says:

> She did marry the best man but now I'm the worst man.
> [Intervewer: What is Alzheimer's disease doing to you?]
> It's making me almost nothing like I was, that's the problem. I have changed like a person dramatically.

For John Bayley, writer and philosopher and husband of novelist and academic Iris Murdoch, the change that occurred in his wife Iris's writing signalled for him a change in Iris's self: 'She seemed to have become a different kind of writer and therefore a different sort of person and that personality change is something you do see in the first stages of Alzheimer's disease' (John Bayley talking about his wife Iris Murdoch on BBC Radio Four on 1 December 2004).

Phrases such as 'She's no longer my mother' or 'the person I knew died years ago' will be familiar to many people who have cared for, or known, people with dementia. They are phrases that capture some family members' experience that their relative with dementia, particularly those with advanced or severe dementia, are seen as no longer the same person they were. Their personness has been eroded by loss of memory. As such, the irretrievable cognitive and functional decline and the loss of self are inextricably linked. We can link this identification of psychological death with social death as it has been observed in a wide variety of people with life-limiting illness. This is discussed in Chapter 6.

A relational view of self

This insistence on cognition as being essential to personhood and self has been criticized by Stephen Post, Tom Kitwood and Julian Hughes among others. Post describes Western society as being 'hyper' cognitive, valuing cognition over other attributes and abilities. Such a society holds the view that without cognition people are non-persons. People lack[1] full moral status[2] as persons when they lack cognition. Adopting a postmodern stance Post (2000ab[3]) argues that such a view ignores many aspects of being human that have nothing to do with cognition. These include emotional and spiritual aspects and relational and aesthetic ones (Post 2000ab).

There are ample narratives from a range of people testifying to the fact that people with dementia retain their essential humanity and connection to their former lives (Ballenger 2006). Gubrium's (2000) ethnographies of carer support group programmes provide evidence that families' experience did not support the philosophical reasoning that self is inevitably lost in dementia. For example, Sorrell (2005) contends that her husband is still a human being who remains the love of her life.

Friedell (2000), who has dementia, sees the diagnosis of dementia as a wake-up call for people to become more their true selves, more like the person they were meant to be. This is reminiscent of Kitwood (1990) who uses the terms experiential and adapted self where the experiential self is the feeling-knowing self, the self which is the source of a person's well-being and relatedness. The adapted or learned self conforms to other people's expectations.

Friedell (2000) suggests that with a life-threatening diagnosis people have the opportunity to be the people they were meant to be. He identifies dementia as part of his life, but says it does not define him. For him, people with dementia retain many abilities, including the ability to feel and relate to other people and to share emotions, especially love. Dementia affords people the opportunity to be sensitive to what is slower and deeper in life, to kindliness and peacefulness (see David quoted in Noyes (2004) in Chapter 2). For one family member, dementia revealed more of the essential qualities of her mother: 'We saw her in her true colours, her strengths and talents were magnified because other things were not there' (Deirdre Downs).

Tappen *et al.* (1999) demonstrates persistence of awareness of self into mid to late dementia in a qualitative study using conversational analysis of 23 people with dementia. They concluded that people are aware of cognitive changes and seek explanations for them. They argue that failure to recognize persistence of the self leads to task-oriented care and low expectations. More recently Surr (2005) provides empirical evidence to support persistence of self when she concludes from her conversations with people with dementia living in residential care settings that the quality of interpersonal relationships is an essential component of the preservation of self. She provides examples of how interactions and relationships can support a person's biography and identity.

There are a variety of overlapping and linked theoretical and philosophical perspectives which broadly support a relational view of self. These include self as situated and embodied; self as socially constructed, self as captured in narrative. We will identify the roots and implications for people with dementia with respect to care of each of these perspectives.

Situated embodied agents

Hughes and colleagues (2006) in a chapter in their edited text, *Dementia: Mind, meaning and person,* use the term personhood when discussing self. For them, personhood is not located in being conscious of one's self but is an inevitable result of being *situated embodied agents.* For them, self is a function of 'our doings and sayings in the world' (Hughes *et al.* 2006: 33) not, as we have shown in Locke's philosophy, a function of our internal 'goings on'. As Hughes *et al.* argue, we:

> need to see self as a situated human being, who engages with the world in a mental and bodily way in agent-like activities, showing (amongst other things) desires, choices, drives, emotions, needs, and attachments.

> (Hughes *et al.* 2006: 35)

Mathews (2006) applies Merleau-Ponty's body subject to people with dementia.[1] He argues that it is not possible to reduce personhood or identity to self-consciousness as such, nor to its continuity (Mathews 2006: 171). A person has not ceased to exist just because they no longer recall personal memories and thus do not have a connected sense of who they are. Rather, Mathews argues, in such a situation a great deal remains. A different idea of what a person is, of what makes a person the individual they are is required. While the person has been diminished by the loss of memory there remains a person who does not rely on these memories, and who still has some memory. Conceding that people with dementia may lose some of their former identity, some elements of the person remain. He goes on to point out that this is what challenges us. It is not that the person is no longer there but that they remain, albeit in a somewhat diminished version (2006: 175). While this may be considered by some to be worse than death he stresses that it is *not* death, as core elements of the person they were continue to exist. People with dementia are not an empty shell with no elements of the personal (Mathews 2006). People with severe dementia retain enough individual identity to be human beings. According to Mathews:

> There survives something of their adult individuality in the habits of behaviour in which it has become 'sedimented' in the course of their development to adulthood and beyond. These characteristic gestures and ways of doing things are what keep alive the sense of the individual they once were, even if the more sophisticated levels of that individuality have been removed.

> (Mathews 2005: 176)

This preservation of the core elements of the person are illustrated in Alan Bennett's description of his Aunty Kathleen 'said to be suffering from arteriosclerosis of the brain' (Bennett 2005: 86):

> Still, despite this formless spate of loquacity she remains recognizably herself, discernible in the flood, those immutable gentilities and components of her talk which have always characterized her (and been such a joke). 'If you follow me Lilian …', 'As it transpired, Walter …', 'Ready to wend my way, if you take my meaning …' So that now, with no story to tell (or half a dozen), she must needs still tell it as genteelly as she has ever done but at five times the speed, her old world politeness detached from any

---

[1] Merleau-Ponty was a twentieth-century French phenomenologist philosopher. He opposed the ideas emanating from John Locke, not least through his formulation of the idea of body-subject. For Merleau-Ponty one's own body is not only a thing, a potential object of study for scientists, but also a permanent condition of experience. See his *Phenomenology of Perception* (1962).

narrative but still whole and hers, bobbing about in ceaseless flood of unmeaning; demented, as she herself might have said, but very nicely spoken. And as with her speech, so it is with her behaviour. Surrounded by the senile and by the wrecks of women as hopelessly, though differently, demented as she is, she still clings to the notion that she is somehow different and superior. Corseted in her immutable gentilities she still contrives to make something special out of her situation and her role in it.

'He'll always give me a smile', she says of an impassive nurse who is handing out the tea. 'I'm his favourite.'

'This is my chair. They'll always put me here because this corner's that bit more select.'

Her life has been made meaningful by frail, fabricated connections, and now, when the proper connections in her brain are beginning to break down, it is this flimsy tissue of social niceties that still holds firm.

In this demented barracks she remains genteel, in circumstances where gentility is hardly appropriate: a man wetting himself; a woman is howling.

'I'll just meander down,' says Aunty, stepping round the widening pool of piss. 'They've stood me in good stead, these shoes'

(Bennett 2005: 87–8)

Self is situated in 'being in the world'. It is embedded in, or exists in relation to, a variety of contexts include biographical, family, community, cultural, and historical. It is these contexts that constitute a person's being. By implication, in order to understand the person their life history and the current context in which they are living must be understood. Actions are only meaningful in a specific narrative and environment (Hughes 2005).

For Hughes

Whilst the person's agency might be whittled away (albeit gestures and behaviour can act as continuing manifestations of agency), if personhood is embedded in the individuals' life history and engagement with others, as well as in his or her bodily form, then it makes sense to still talk of the person even in severe dementia.

(Hughes 2001: 90)

It is possible to identify ways in which people with dementia are embodied and situated. Kontos's (2004) ethnographic study in a long-term care setting argues that selfhood persists even with severe dementia. It is argued that selfhood is an embodied dimension of human existence. Evidence is presented of people with dementia interacting 'meaningfully with the world through their embodied way of being-in-the-world' (Kontos 2004: 829). Similarly, as described in chapter two, Phinney and Chesla (2003) describe the 'lived body' in dementia, illustrating how the brain's workings are expressed through the body, and is manifest in everyday habits and practices.

From the narrative perspective, self is constantly changing, adapting to new experiences that are assimilated into the life story. Thus, while dementia may change self, as would other major life changes like marriage, having children, divorce, bereavement, self is retained. Living with chronic illness requires a narrative reconstruction such that a new story is told, one that integrates illness into the life story (Holstein and Cole 1996, cited by Lyman 1998) (we consider narrative theories of self in more detail below). For Lyman (1998), who adopted a phenomenological perspective in her fieldwork with people with dementia attending day centres, this allows for a recreation of meaning and an affirmation of the changed self:

> We are challenged to find ways to recognize their personhood as they become less able to articulate their own perspective, and to support their struggle to create meaning while living with Alzheimer's disease.

> (Lyman 1998: 56)

Lyman demonstrated that people with dementia incorporate the experience of having dementia into their identity and they re-create meaning to maintain self. She describes how people with dementia attending the day centre integrate dementia in to their life story. Lyman (1998) is interested in the experience of illness and not disease progression. For her:

> The *self is reconstituted* by people who live with disability, incorporating illness and impairment in to new narratives about one's life, emphasizing continuity rather than loss: 'I haven't changed much, really, but I have to accept what I can't do any more' (her italics).

> (Lyman 1998: 53)

Welie (2004), too, in describing a constitutive versus destructive model of dementia, describes how changes associated with dementia are integrated into one's self. She describes these as being of the same order as change associated with getting old or getting married or becoming widowed. All such changes alter us. There is not a self that is distinct and hiding from an outside attacker. Rather, there is a self who changes, adjusts, adapts and assimilates dementia into their being. In this way, the person continues to have needs and wishes, goals and desires even if they cannot articulate or defend them. The person is an active agent, responding to the world they have found themself in, developing new interests and needs. This active interest in, and response to, the world is evident in Bayley's (1998) description of Iris Murdoch enjoying watching the children's TV programme *Telly Tubbies*, even though the image of her doing this is at odds with her status as a formidable and complex thinker.

Social constructionist accounts

A second, yet closely related, view of the self is that self is socially constructed. From a social constructionist perspective the degree of change in self in dementia is as much attributed to the person's social world – at micro and macro levels – as to the neurological disease itself. While social constructionists argue that self may be changed by dementia, much of this change is attributed to how we interact with the person at interpersonal, societal and political levels. For example, the language used to describe people living with dementia, 'the living dead', influences the manner in which interpersonal interaction occurs. The social constructionist approach also underlines the complexity of the concept defined as 'self'. Here Sabat's (2005) presentation of three aspects of selfhood is of particular interest and this is described below. An understanding of the self as being constructed in relationship to, and with, others was postulated, most famously by George Herbert Mead (1932). As we have shown, there are elements of social constructionist accounts in situated embodied agent accounts of self.

Kitwood (1997a), Sabat (2001) and others provide a social constructionist account of dementia. Those around the person contribute to their personhood, self is not a given property of the person, a function of cognition or personality, but is created or diminished in interaction and relationships. Personhood is shaped in the caring relationship (Kitwood 1997, Woods 1999, 2001).

The implications of this approach to self for people with dementia are far reaching. If self is constructed in relationship with others then the other assumes an important role in the maintenance of self for people with dementia. It is the situatedness of self that is of most interest to social constructionists. Kitwood (1994) uses the term personhood when describing self in dementia.

Kitwood (1993a, b) argues that personhood does not exist as an abstract attribution but is created by our actions and interactions. For him these maintain or diminish the personhood of people with dementia. Kitwood (1998) identified 12 kinds of interactions that maintain personhood and 17 kinds that undermine it, providing operational definitions of each. He called those which maintained personhood 'positive enhancers' and, together, these constituted what he called 'positive person work' (Box 4.1).

He called those interactions which undermined personhood 'personal detractors', which together constituted a 'malignant social psychology' (Kitwood and Bredin 1992a, b) (Box 4.2). These were malignant because they were damaging to personhood and self and led to the depersonalization of people with dementia.

For Kitwood, a good care environment was one where there was positive person work free of malignant social psychology. In this way Kitwood places

Box 4.1 Postive person work: positive enhancers

- recognition
- negotiation
- collaboration
- play
- celebration
- relaxation
- validation
- holding
- timalation (sensuous or sensual interaction providing contact, reassurance and pleasure)
- creation
- giving
- facilitation

(Kitwood 1998: 27–9)

the onus for loss of self on the other people in a person's life. People with dementia, as we have discussed, are at risk of being depersonalized, as being seen as a task to be 'done to' rather than a person to 'be with', as one 'does for'.

Sabat (2001) coined the term 'malignant social positioning', which, resonant with Kitwood's malignant social psychology, refers to an experience that assaults the personhood of individuals with dementia. Such assaults have been justified on the grounds that people with dementia lack awareness (Downs 2005).

Sabat proposes that there are different aspects of selfhood: Self 1, 2 and 3 (Sabat and Harré 1992). Self 1 is the self of personal identity, of being a singularity and having one and the same point of view over time. It is expressed through indexical pronouns such as 'I' and 'me'. Self 2 is the self of physical and mental attributes such as height and sense of humour. These attributes can be viewed as being positive or negative. Self 3 is the multiplicity of social identities that we construct with the cooperation of others. These include our self as partner, as worker, as patient. Self 3 is vulnerable in dementia because if others only see us in a socially devalued role, for example as a patient, this limits our social identity. Loss of this kind of self has its roots in the social world, not in neuropathology (Sabat 2006). Such 'malignant positioning' is not unique to

Box 4.2 Malignant social psychology – personal detractors

- treachery
- disempowerment
- infantilization
- intimidation
- labelling
- stigmatization
- outpacing
- invalidation
- banishment
- objectification
- ignoring
- imposition
- withholding
- accusation
- disruption
- mockery
- disparagement

(Kitwood 1998: 29–30)

dementia and is also seen for people with any psychiatric diagnosis (Sayce 1999). Sabat *et al.* (2004) describe how the person with dementia requires the 'cooperation' of others in order to 'construct a valued social identity'. They note that often the only identity permitted the person with dementia is that of 'dysfunctional patient'. Such malignant positioning leads to social embarrass-ment and a diminished sense of self worth. Sabat *et al.* (2004) distinguish between the capacity for recall and recognition. They argue that people retain implicit memory such that they may have a memory of an event without being conscious of it. Loss of self, they argue, is due to the perspective of others and not to actual loss within the person.

'It is in the social dynamics of everyday life beyond the neuropathological processes in their brains that people with dementia can be supported in, or experience assaults on, their personhood' (Sabat 2006b: 298). An example of how difficult it can be to avoid 'positioning' can be found in the BBC Radio 4 programme which we cited earlier, one in which David Whitcombe and his family were discussing the effect his Alzheimer's disease had had on their lives. These are David's wife's words:

> Because we can't talk so much together and discuss things, it changes the whole rela-tionship. We used to banter a lot, didn't we? And joke with each other a lot. It's all gone. The relationship is very much a carer and a patient rather than a husband and a wife, which is very sad. But at the same time you make the most of what you've got left, you have to. Some evenings we try to have a chat, but I get frustrated.

> (BBC Radio Four 8 November 2005)

Positioning can be seen in other situations too. Bogdan and Taylor (1989) demonstrated that non-disabled people construct, or fail to construct, the humanity of severely disabled children. They argued that whether a disabled child was viewed as a person or not had little to do with the extent of their impairment and more to do with the perspective of the non-disabled person (Bogdan and Taylor 1989).

For Kitwood (1997a) both the potential for exclusion and exclusion itself serves as the greatest threat to quality of life, far exceeding the challenges of living with cognitive impairment per se. Lyman's work supports this position. People with anticipated and diagnosed dementia are aware of how others view them and the potential threat dementia poses to relationships (Lyman 1998; Moniz-Cook et al. 2006). Lyman's (1998) phenomenological study in day centres demon-strated that people with dementia were aware of how others viewed and treated them. It was often the reactions of others, rather than cognitive impairment per se, which made life with dementia difficult. Box 4.3 provides an example.

Box 4.3 Mum

On the way to the airport
We stopped for a coffee in a hotel lounge
Mum looked dishevelled
A man kept staring over at her
She turned to me and said
'you'd think he'd never seen a person in his life.'

Murna Downs

Kitwood (1997a) argues that a concern with order and the elevation of rationality to a pre-eminent position has resulted in people with dementia being positioned outside the 'people club'. For him, 'cultures are underpinned by psychological defences, these are likely to be particularly strong when the issue is as threatening as dementia' (Kitwood 1997a: 137).[2] This is not unlike the historical sequestration observed in the care of older people (e.g. Townsend 1962) and it also resonates with the sequestration of the dying, a subject we will return to in Chapter 6. Kitwood (1997a) described the situation of many people with demenitia and people who are dying as illustrating that 'one can be a human being, and yet not be acknowledged as a person' (Kitwood 1997a: Kitwood and Bredin 1992a, b).

Bogdan and Taylor (1989) describe four ways that have been identified to counter this positioning and dehumanization of people with profound disabilities:

1. attributing thinking to the other;

2. seeing the individuality in the other;

3. viewing the other as reciprocating; and

4. defining social place for the other.

Much of Bogdan and Taylor's discussion of the situation of people with profound disabilities can be used to illuminate the circumstance of people with dementia. This requires that we

> Recognise people with severe disabilities as 'someone like me', that is, as having the essential qualities to be defined as a fellow human being. Disability is viewed as secondary to the person's humaneness.
>
> (Bogdan and Taylor 1989: 146)

For Kitwood, the alternative construction is one illuminated in Buber's identification of the *I–Thou* mode of relating, making contact with the pure being of another, with no distinct purpose save the affirmation and confirmation of personhood. This is contrasted to the 'I–It' encounter that is characteristic

---

2 This quote locates Kitwood in a tradition of radical philosophy that includes Freud and Foucault. The former is present in the style of this quote, the latter in the way that he maps how people with dementia have been approached historically – see Kitwood (1997a: 42–5). In this he is on similar ground to Foucault who argued that the pursuit of rationality is implemented through segregation and the subjugation of the non-rational, first via moral correction and then by medical categorization and treatment (see Foucault 1967). Foucault's subjects include the imprisoned, the sick and the insane. We have considered Foucault's relevance for our argument in Chapter 1.

of much of our interaction. This latter encounter exhibits coolness, an information-getting objectivity, an instrumentality, and an engagement without commitment (Buber 1970; see Small *et al.* 2006). Kitwood proposes three characteristics that are necessary if one wishes to enhance 'personhood':

1. a recognition of uniqueness,

2. an acceptance of subjectivity; and

3. an acceptance of relatedness (from Kitwood 1997a).

All three characteristics call into question established tenets of modernity, all are consistent with postmodernity.

Narrative theories of self

Proponents of narrative theories of self argue that people are narrative beings, selves are constructed through narrative, through stories. These stories include stories people tell about themselves and stories others tell about them. People with dementia are at risk of others assuming they do not have a narrative, or if they do, of it not being understandable. Consequently, if people are narrative beings and are seen as having no narrative, or no accessible narrative, this leads to the conclusion that there is no self with dementia.

The use of the concept of narrative for people with severe dementia can at first seem problematic (Baldwin 2005). Given that people with dementia can have difficulty finding the right words to describe something, and as the disease progresses have difficulty producing words at all, how then can narrative theories of self be applied to them? At least two ways in which dementia compromises 'the narrative enterprise' have been identified (Baldwin 2005). First, cognitive impairment may make it difficult for people to construct a coherent or recognizable narrative. Secondly, and no less important, the stigma associated with dementia may make others less likely to take the trouble to make sense of their narrative. As protagonists and as accompaniers to the primary narrative and narrator other people can maintain, challenge, disrupt, strengthen or hinder another person's story. A person's apparent loss of narrative can erroneously be attributed to their loss of self rather than to the limitations of current narrative theory to incorporate the experience of cognitive impairment. In this way people become 'narratively dispossessed'. Narrative theory and practice combine to deny the possibility of narrativity to people with dementia.

Baldwin argues that there is a need to reconceptualize the nature and role of narrative. He argues that there are ways to enhance a person's 'narrative integrity and agency', to facilitate the construction of meaningful narratives for people with dementia, and for others who are similarly dispossessed for example those with severe mental illness (Baldwin 2006a: 218). The task he identifies is to mobilize meta narratives on the part of others to understand, contain or manage those who are at risk of being narratively dispossessed.

Baldwin cites the example of Hogeway, a residential setting, as a place where, through the manipulation of the physical and social environment, narrative continuity is supported. Hogeway has different environments to reflect the different lifestyles represented by the people living there (Notter *et al.* 2004). For example, there is an area devoted to farming where former farmers live. Likewise, an area of Clonakilty Hospital has been designed to reflect the lifestyle lived in this rural part of Ireland, with bread-making a daily event and the smell of a peat fire pervading the atmosphere. Such narrative continuity is also the aim of biographical and life story work (Bruce 1998). In this way biography is not disrupted (Bury 1982) but maintained.

Two kinds of narratives have been identified amongst people recently diagnosed with dementia (Clare 2003). 'Self-maintaining' strategies have as their aim maintaining the prior sense of self by viewing dementia as a normal experience, as a natural part of ageing. 'Self-adjusting' narratives, on the other hand, acknowledge the changes that dementia brings and integrate them into one's sense of self. Such ways of adapting to dementia are influenced by how people see dementia, the illness representation they are working with (Harman and Clare 2006). Narrative theories of self fit well within a postmodern approach. First, they allow for multiple realities and selves over time. Secondly, they allow the person to be their own expert as to who they are at this point in time. Thirdly, they take as valid the person with dementia's perspective, however at odds it is with other views. Fourthly, they accept that accounts of both lives and self do not have to be linear and progressive but can be jumbled up much as they are for people with dementia.

In this section we have presented self as constituted by cognition, self as constituted in relation to others and to social context and self as constituted in and through narrative. We have argued that self exists independently of cognition. Social constructionists argue that self is formed and maintained in relationship to others. Accounts of self from the perspective of situated embodied agents argue that self is intrinsic to being embodied. Self also exists in the stories told by a person and by people about a person. We will now examine the concept of autonomy for people with dementia, drawing on these approaches to how self is constituted and maintained.

Autonomy

Having considered the extent to which the person with dementia retains personhood, we now turn to examine the appropriateness of autonomy as a guiding principle in the care of people with dementia, particularly towards the end of life (Nolan *et al.* 2004; McCormack 2001; Robinson *et al.* 2005a). We will look at the problems that an uncritical acceptance of autonomy poses for people with dementia and their families and how these might be overcome. We will argue for an ethic of care which does not privilege autonomy over connectedness and over caring communities.

Autonomy is a value held dear in contemporary Western society. Respect for autonomy is implicit in the Council of Europe's 2003 Convention for the Protection of Human Rights and Fundamental Freedoms. Respect for autonomy has been described as the leading guiding principle in Western bioethics (Beauchamp and Childress 1994) and contemporary health and social care (Welie 2004). Autonomy, and the promotion of independence, are enshrined in the UK government's Department of Health (1992) *Patients' charter*. A concern with autonomy and independence underlie many approaches to improving care for older people. The recent Mental Capacity Act in the UK (HM Government 2005) reinforces a person's right to make decisions and to be assumed to be able to do so unless proven otherwise (Table 4.1).

The growth of consumerism in the 1970s and 1980s contributed to a more critical stance being taken towards a prevailing paternalism in the health and social care system. The patient was recast as consumer. This elevated a concern with voice and choice – the patient should be able to express their preferences and should have their views of services listened to. They should have some measure of choice over when, where and how they were cared for. This idea of health and social care as a commodity and the patient as consumer coexisted with a recognition that the development and increasing use of medical technologies was prompting a need to consider patients' rights in the context of,

Table 4.1 Mental Capacity Act: the principles

The following principles apply for the purposes of this Act.

(1) A person must be assumed to have capacity unless it is established that he lacks capacity.

(2) A person is not to be treated as unable to make a decision unless all practicable steps to help him to do so have been taken without success.

(3) A person is not to be treated as unable to make a decision merely because he makes an unwise decision.

(4) An act done, or decision made, under this Act for or on behalf of a person who lacks capacity must be done, or made, in his best interests.

(5) Before the act is done, or the decision is made, regard must be had to whether the purpose for which it is needed can be as effectively achieved in a way that is less restrictive of the person's rights and freedom of action.

From www.opsi.gov.uk, accessed 13 November 2006.

for example, intensive care, life support and transplantation (Kissell 2004). We will examine in more detail in Chapter 5 the changing emphasis of the health and social care system in the context of wider social and political change.

This emphasis on individuals and choice can be identified in policies issued over the last few years related to both palliative care and care for older people (Froggatt 2005).

In relation to the provision of cancer care (which at this time subsumed palliative care) The Policy Framework for Commissioning Cancer Services, known as the 'Calman-Hine Report' included as a general principles that:

> The development of cancer services should be patient centred and should take account of patient', families' and carers' views and preferences as well as those of professionals involved in cancer care.
>
> (Expert Advisory Group on Cancer 1995: 6)

This statement frames choice with respect to the development of services, rather than choices about an individual's care. The NHS Cancer Plan (Department of Health 2000) and the associated document 'Improving Supportive and Palliative Care for Adults with Cancer' (National Institute for Clinical Excellence 2004) is more explicitly focused on individuals and their choices. It states that individuals should 'have their voice heard, to be valued for their knowledge and skills and to be able to exercise real choice about treatments and services' (National Institute for Clinical Excellence 2004: 15).

More specifically in terms of palliative care in the UK, the House of Commons Health Committee considered palliative care and produced a report outlining its considerations (House of Commons Health Committee 2004). A key area of concern was the issue of choice in palliative care. By now, though, the focus of the choice debate is on the place of care and of dying. The summary for this report begins:

> Currently, around 56% of people die in hospital, 20% at home, 20% in nursing or residential homes and 4% in hospices. Yet surveys show that the majority of people would prefer to be supported to die in their own homes.
>
> (House of Commons Health Committee 2004: 3)

Alongside these developments within palliative care, there have been policy initiatives affecting care for older people that illustrate a similar trend of increasing emphasis on choice. The National Service Framework for Older People (Department of Health 2001a), launched in March 2001, aimed to improve and standardize the quality of care for older people. Eight areas of care are addressed and Standard 2, 'Person Centred Care', puts choice at the centre: 'NHS and social care services treat older people as individuals and enable them to make choices about their own care' (Department of Health 2001a: 23).

There is also specific reference to this choice making about care at the end of life in a section titled 'Dignity in end-of-life care':

> This emphasis on choice with respect to service provision, and more specifically on choice about place of care until death, is problematic when its assumptions are applied to people with dementia. For example, whilst evidence is presented that shows that people when asked would prefer to die at home, this research is usually undertaken well in advance of their condition deteriorating and of their being an immediate need for end of life care. This sort of antecedent autonomy is problematic in dementia not least because the communication problems that accompany advanced dementia mean that it is difficult to ascertain if the person's preference has changed.

Challenges dementia poses autonomy

To be capable of autonomous acts one has to be competent to make decisions, that is to acquire, retain and critically appraise information, free of outside interference or impairment. While a diagnosis of dementia does not automatically mean a person is no longer capable of making decisions, as the condition progresses, most would agree that a person with severe dementia is no longer autonomous in the sense of being able to make rational, deliberate and explicit decisions. Several solutions have been proposed to address this dilemma. Two of these work within the broad concept of autonomy and include antecedent autonomy, where the decisions executed by the person prior to developing dementia hold for the person who is living with dementia, and embodied autonomy, where a person's current behaviour and actions are seen as reflecting their will and their self.

Autonomy refers to the right of a person to decide for him/herself, to have control over what happens. There are many definitions of autonomy but Hofland (1994), citing Collopy, suggests that they all centre around the idea of self determination and freedom, control of decision-making free of outside interference (Agich 1993; Collopy 1988). Research from social gerontology and social psychology demonstrating the link between control over one's life and well-being, suggests that autonomy, like security, is a basic human need (Zarit and Braungart 2006).

In this section, we will argue that conventional definitions of autonomy risk excluding people with dementia and that solutions which have been put in place to cater for loss of self, primarily focusing on antecedent autonomy, risk violating the present self. We argue that the capacity to exercise autonomy, like understandings of the self, is enhanced or diminished by the behaviour, practices and policies of professionals, family members and society as well as by the cognitive changes of dementia.

A word of caution about autonomy and dementia

Consistent with the UK Mental Capacity Act (HM Government 2005), a diagnosis of Alzheimer's disease does not necessarily mean that the person lacks competence to make decisions (Werner 2006; Zarit and Braungart, 2006). If diagnosis occurs early, people are able to articulate feelings and preferences and concerns (Woods 1999) – they do not need someone to talk for them. By adopting the sorts of communication strategies and attitudes promoted by Sabat (1991a, b, 1999), Small (2003), Small *et al.* (2004) and Whitlatch *et al.* (2006), people can answer questions posed.

Sabat (2005) warns against the danger of 'positioning' the person as incapable of making decisions on the basis of their having a diagnosis of dementia. Assuming that people with dementia are unable to communicate in a meaningful way invalidates their part in decision-making and obscures areas of resource and competence (Woods 1999). Even if people with dementia are deemed by a court as incompetent to make decisions about certain aspects of their life, they still retain capacities. These include the capacity for meaning-making and experiencing emotions such as shame and embarrassment. If people with dementia are positioned as lacking awareness of the meaning of a situation, the opportunity to understand their behaviour is lost. Sabat (2005) argues that people with dementia retain cognitive abilities, including implicit and long-term memory, which make them able to make decisions about certain aspects of their lives; they should not be denied this opportunity.

People with dementia are not all the same. People with mild to moderate dementia can express preferences about their care and preferred living circumstances. They consistently report preferences and choices in daily matters (Feinberg and Whitlatch 2001; Mozley *et al.* 1999) and most people express a desire to be involved in decision-making (see Zarit and Braungart 2006 for a review of studies on this topic). For people with more profound cognitive impairment who are less able to verbally articulate their wishes and preferences, alternative strategies can be used. These include observing and interpreting subtle behavioural cues (Brooker 2005; McCormack 2001) and gathering information about a person's past and present preferences and reactions (Clarke *et al.* 1993; Hepburn *et al.* 1997).

It is well recognized that it is difficult to determine the extent to which a person is competent or incompetent. While in the past a doctor's letter could deem someone to be lacking in competence, today in the UK and US it must be established by a court (Zarit and Braungart 2006). More recently, a distinction has been made between various levels and domains of competence. It is now recognized that competency is multidimensional, fluctuates over time and can vary to the extent that one can be competent in some areas and not in others (Zarit and Braungart 2006). It is clear that competency is not a zero-sum concept.

Competence is better thought of as representing a continuum (Hofland 1994). Perhaps autonomy can be considered in the same way. While people with dementia may not be able to decide how to invest their life savings, they may well be able to express a preference for which care assistant helps them undress. Moody (1988) argues that people with dementia should participate in decisions about their care as competency is not global but functionally specific. Nevertheless, as the condition progresses people with dementia will have difficulty meeting the criteria that sees them as autonomous individuals as set down by Beauchamp and Childress (1994).

Proposed solutions for the challenge of autonomy

Antecedent autonomy

One position adopted in the face of the eventual loss of capacity to make decisions is referred to as antecedent autonomy. This refers to the practice whereby decisions made by the person antecedent (prior) to their being deemed incompetent to decide are upheld. In this way decisions are made antecedent to the destruction of self (Welie 2004). The concept of antecedent autonomy attempts to address the difficulty inherent in a cognitive-based autonomy by referring to the 'then' and the 'now' self, thus distinguishing between the person 'then' – i.e. before cognitive loss and disruption – and the person 'now', i.e. with cognitive impairment.

Antecedent autonomy most commonly takes the form of advance directives (Welie 2004). Advance directives can be:

- A living will or set of instructions for health care

- Substituted judgment or power of attorney where someone is identified to speak on one's behalf once one has become incompetent. This defines on what basis they are to make decisions and, if not specified, then to use substituted judgement – to step into the person with dementia's shoes. Such an approach does not resolve the question 'which person with dementia, the person now or the person then?'

Welie (2004) describes how, from this perspective, advance directives (or living wills) can be likened to financial wills. They serve to direct someone's affairs when they are no longer around. In the case of advance directives, the person is assumed to be gone. As such advance directives are seen to be antecedent to one's own destruction. They serve the purpose of maintaining a narrative continuity.

This fits well with a cognitive view of self for, as we have seen above, in this view there is the person or self before cognitive impairment and the person after. For example, Hope (1994) cited by Hughes (2001) argues that 'a man before and after dementia is a different person' (Hughes 2001: 89).

We will now look at how advance directives may assist with decision-making as to whether to treat or withhold treatment at the end of life. Alzheimer Europe support the use of advance directives in decision-making as they respect 'previously expressed wishes' (Alzheimer Europe 2005). Both US and UK Alzheimer's Societies advocate the use of advance directives regarding treatment decisions at the end of life. They recommend that such discussions should take place soon after diagnosis while the person still retains the capacity to make decisions about future health care for themself. In the US the Alzheimer's Association notes that 'all efforts at life extension in the advanced stage of Alzheimer's creates burdens and avoidable suffering for patients who could otherwise live out the remainder of their lives in greater comfort and peace'.

The Alzheimer's Society of England, Wales and Northern Ireland recommends that invasive technologies, including antibiotics, should be avoided. This should be recommended to people with dementia and their families soon after initial diagnosis. In their view early discussion about peaceful dying should occur. The assumption for both these societies is that early and ongoing consultation between a person with dementia and family members and health professionals is critical if a person is to achieve genuine shared decision-making (Alzheimer's Society 2007b).

A variety of criticisms have made of the use of antecedent autonomy as the solution to the problem of autonomy for people with dementia (for a review, see Rich 1998). These include:

1. that antecedent autonomy provides us with a 'disrupted' view of the person and does little to affirm the contemporary personhood of people with dementia;

2. that antecedent autonomy is morally problematic;

3. that advance directives as a vehicle for antecedent autonomy are hard to ensure on a practical level.

We will now discuss these in turn.

There are those who argue that, while intuitively appealing in its simplicity, the use of advance directives provides us with a 'disrupted' view of what it means to be a person with dementia (Baldwin 2006a). It fails to attend to the imperceptible changes that characterize living with dementia. These afford people the opportunity to prepare for, and negotiate, 'a less disruptive narrative of transformation' (Baldwin 2006b: 220). As already argued in the constitutive account of self, dementia can become integrated into one's narrative and hence into one's sense of self (Lyman 1998; Welie 2004).

Consequently, the solutions of advance directives and substituted judgments do little to affirm the contemporary personhood of the person with dementia. Relying on antecedent autonomy thus risks discounting the person as experiencing and expressing self in their present reality (Welie 2004) as when the 'then' self may be diminished or eroded, we can work with the 'now' self. For Welie (2004) the problem with advance directives are that they 'can entail a serious violation of the patient's intrinsic dignity because they tend to deny the condition from which the patient is suffering now and for the remainder of his or her life' (Welie 2004: 165).

Some writers argue that advance directives are morally problematic for two reasons. First, they have no moral authority because the person is a different person to who they were when they made the directive (Rich 1998). Furthermore, for Rich (1998), they fail to meet the requirements of informed consent regarding treatment, as treatments may later become available that were not available at the time of the directive (Rich 1998). Secondly, while advance directives offer a route to honouring people's wishes, reliance on them puts us at risk of taking responsibility away from concerned others for what happens to the person (Kissell 2004).

On a more practical level, advance directives are problematic as they assume a health care system which engages in early diagnosis. As we have shown in Chapter 3, the delay in diagnosing dementia until late in the condition has, on a practical level, made the uptake of advance directives problematic. Plus we have noted the lack of services and supports available to people recently diagnosed with dementia.

Embodied autonomy

Embodied autonomy is based on the premise that people with severe dementia retain selfhood and that it is experienced and expressed through the body (Dekkers 2004). This links to the concept of self as a situated embodied agent which we discussed earlier. Rather than viewing behaviour from a biomedical Cartesian dualist perspective, as something separate from, but under the control of, the self, embodied autonomy is built on the premise that bodily expressions tell us something about the person's wishes and the person's self. Behaviour becomes the expression of will and also a remnant of what we may have previously identified as rational autonomy.

A focus on embodiment underlines that people with dementia, like all people, are semiotic beings – they act on the basis of the meaning they make of their world (Sabat and Harré 1994, Sabat 2006b). People with dementia 'act from a point of view and with a purpose' (Hughes 2001: 88). Such a view provides an alternative interpretation of challenging behaviour. It can be argued that there is a relationship between autonomy and agency, and that 'challenging behaviour' is a manifestation of agency or autonomy or of both (McCormack 2001; Graneheim *et al.* 2001). If it is assumed that behaviour is the bodily enactment of will, then it becomes possible to promote autonomy, and to focus on enhancing quality of life. For example, if someone is continually going to the door wanting to leave the care setting, one could accept the obvious and conclude that they no longer want to be where they are. Equally, if someone insists on going home (when they are now permanent residents of a nursing home or indeed in their own home) this could be interpreted as a clear evaluative statement that this environment – whether it be the entire building or the part they happen to be in at that time – does not feel like home to them. It does not fulfill the criteria of home, perhaps the most important being that one might expect to feel a sense of belonging, ease and comfort.

One can only make sense of a person's behaviour by examining the context in which it arises. That includes the biographical, environmental, interpersonal, cultural and historical context. For Lyman (1998) viewing behavioural expressions as 'troublesome' or 'challenging' is a result of seeking a biomedical explanation for behaviour rather than a contextual one. For her many of these 'problems' are better understood as having social and environmental origins rather than biomedical. Stokes' *Challenging behaviour in dementia: a person-centred approach* (2000) provides guidance as to how to adopt such an analytical approach to practice. As discussed in Chapter 3, viewing behaviour as acts of will and, thus, a form of embodied autonomy stands in stark contrast to the neuropsychiatric view of dementia where behavioural symptoms are seen as inevitable consequences of brain disease.

Beyond autonomy – recognition of the need for a different ethic of care

Respect for the principle of autonomy has played an important role in giving control of bodies back to the individuals and away from medical power, but principlist ethics perpetuates a dualism between subject and body and person and community. Considering the challenges raised by dementia requires us to engage critically with the principles on which Western bioethics are based (Cassell 2004). Our presentation, in this chapter, of self as embodied and situated, self from a social constructivist perspective and narrative perspectives offers an alternative reading captured as a relational sense of self. This different approach to self necessitates a comprehensive, integrated, situated, embodied and relational ethic, an ethic that views human beings as more than rational agents seeking control over their body, disconnected from relationships and community.

When autonomy is the driving principle we risk placing the person in a position of opposition to their families or, at the very least, as though they are independent of their relationships (Kissell 2004). Indeed a health care system that is exclusively guided by a concern for autonomy fails to recognize the contributions of the many different parties involved, including health care professionals (Nolan *et al.* 2004). In palliative care the unit of care is not the individual in isolation from the family and community, rather it is the person in relationship to others (Kissell 2004; ten Have 2004). Palliative care recognizes the person's essential embeddedness in relationship and family. It is this embodiment and situatedness which constitutes people as human beings. A palliative care approach might be identified as being more concerned with relationships than with autonomy.

The embodied and situated approach to self makes the question of whether it is the same person or a different person early and late in the dementia journey irrelevant (Kissell 2004). For people with dementia, as for people at the end of life, the capacity for rational decision-making is not the only route to respect and dignity. Rather, one's vulnerability within a family or community can be a source of dignity through an essential connection to others.

An ethic of care has been developed by feminist theorists in the last 20 years (Gilligan 1982; Noddings 1984, 2002) which can trace its roots to Aristotle. Such an ethic recognizes that caring is basic to human life, that by their very nature, people are caring beings. People like to be cared for and to care. Caring is a state of being in relation to others characterized by receptivity and openness to the other's experience, relatedness, motivational displacement and reciprocity. To be cared for and to care are natural parts of shared humanity (Nussbaum 2004). Care occurs within interpersonal relationships; interpersonal relationships are care. For these theorists, ethics is not abstract or objective or impersonal but an inevitable part of interpersonal relationships and central to morality. It requires emotional involvement, not detachment, in a context where emotions provide us with information.

Kitwood (1998) recognized the need for attention to be given to an ethic of care and an ethics of justice, and described an education programme designed to achieve this end. He made a compelling argument for promoting moral and professional development of care workers, a term he used to refer to all those who work with people with dementia. He stressed that too much attention was paid to the big health care decisions and not enough to the ethics of process and ethics of context, by which he meant the ethical issues present in how people relate to each other in everyday life (Kitwood 1998). As dementia makes people 'exceptionally dependent on others' both physically and psychologically, he argued the need for an ethic of care that took account of everyday interactions (Kitwood 1998: 23).

We have already introduced links between this aspect of Kitwood's approach and the approach of Buber who distinguished I–It and I–Thou relationships. An ethic of care based on the I and Thou interactions or on *being with* has its limitations when applied to people with dementia (Small *et al.* 2006). This ethic emphasizes people being 'side by side'. Such an emphasis on reciprocity may disadvantage people with dementia, who may have difficulty playing their part in the mutual exchange of solidarity. Bauman's *being for* provides an elegant solution to this problem: 'Being for the Other before being with the Other is the first reality of the self, a starting point rather than a product of society' (Bauman 1993: 13).

This interest in the ethic of *being for* sits well with others who critique the priority given to autonomy over alternative guiding ethics (Hertogh 2004a; Nolan *et al.* 2004). Small *et al.* (2006) argue that if a reliance on autonomy as the guiding principle in care of people with dementia may well result in situations of inadequate care. For a person whose key concerns are to feel safe and cared for, an emphasis on autonomy is not helpful (Hertogh 2004b). Like Kitwood, Ignatieff argues that meeting a person's psychological needs is of paramount concern, amongst them their needs for love, security and belonging (Ignatieff 1984: 13–14).

Thus we come full circle, and alongside a postmodern view of dementia we promote a postmodern view of an ethical approach to care for people with dementia (Small *et al.* 2006). Such an approach emphasizes *being for* the other, whatever their capacity for independence or autonomy and opens up the possibility of a world where 'people matter as individuals, for who they are and not what they can do' (Small *et al.* 2006: 386).

Conclusion

In this chapter we have argued that self persists throughout the experience of living with dementia. We support this argument with reference to situated embodied agent, social constructionist and narrative accounts of self. Furthermore, we provide illustrations from personal testimony and literature in support of this view. We then argue that if self persists despite cognitive impairment, cognition-based autonomy may not be the most useful guiding ethical principle on which to base care for people with dementia. Instead, we argue for an ethic of care that recognizes the importance of our relatedness to one another and our natural tendency to be cared for and to care.

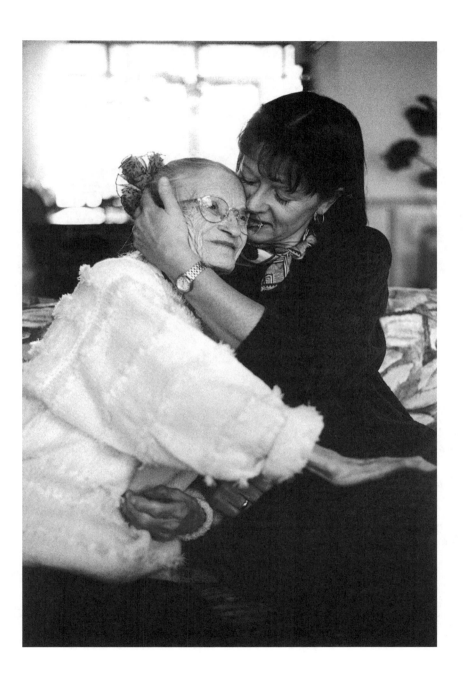

Chapter 5

Quality of care and quality of life

And what is good, Phaedrus,
And what is not good-
Need we ask anyone to tell us these things?
Robert M Pirsig, (Zen and the Art of Motorcycle
Maintenance 1974)

Introduction

In this chapter our aims are modest. We want to focus on one aspect of the system world, a concern to deliver high-quality services. We will examine the assumptions that underpin quality and will argue that these assumptions result in limited benefits for people with dementia. Quality is an attractive subject to choose because it has become important in considering both the structure and process of service delivery and, when oriented to quality of life concerns, has become a widely acceptable outcome measure for those conditions where the intention is not cure. Further, it is a 'hurrah word', something that, superficially, people should be in favour of. Our approach in this chapter will be to say that even when the intentions of care providers are good there are problems in the service models developed because of the assumptions around which they are built.

We will begin this chapter with a consideration of the term quality and look at how it has evolved in the context of the UK National Health Service. There are different ways quality has been approached and we will list some of the more important models and initiatives. However, there is also a case to be made that quality might not be a good system goal to pursue and we will introduce the key arguments in this debate. We will then go on to examine quality of care and the ways it has been conceptualized and measured. This will involve considering the role of audit. We will seek to identify what is 'good care'. In so doing we will present the ways in which care for people with dementia currently addresses, or fails to address, their end of life concerns. We then turn to a consideration of quality of life as an outcome in palliative care and in dementia care. There have been many attempts to devise ways of measuring quality of life with a view to using these measures to evaluate services in chronic and end of life care. These attempts include complex scales addressing functional capacities and they include attempts to access the subjective experience of living with illness. We will examine the connections between a focus on quality of care and quality of life, problematizing the assumption that improving what we define from outside as good quality of care enhances the subjective judgement of quality of life. We will ask if, and in what way, care providers can help a person maintain a good quality of life and what this might mean for people with dementia.

Hence, the focus is on how the system world shapes the life-world, how the limitations that result are manifested and how they can be struggled with. We will present system world assumptions but also bear in mind the voice of person with dementia or the person with palliative care needs. The 'insider' views of these people can be contrasted with what the system world offers as objective or analytic knowledge. This sort of knowledge relates to perceptions of need and how to recognize if need has been met. The system/life-world distinction is similar to an approach that distinguishes between insider and outsider views, between emic and etic accounts (Agar 1996; McNamara 2004). The challenge for prioritizing the emic is that the etic is supported by systems of power which structure context and shape meaning. That is, the parameters of the possible as seen from the emic is defined by the etic.

This distinction between different ways of seeing the same thing presents us with two challenges, one analytic and the other practical. What is understood as rational, as objective and as scientific (the etic) changes over time. Rationality is not fixed, new domains of rationality are constituted. Yesterday's rationality is relegated to the status of, at best, mistaken knowledge and at worst superstition by the advances of today. The history of ideas has not stopped with our present state of knowledge and we can be confident that in the future we will look back on what we now assume as scientific rationality in the same way. One of the writers who has interrogated the way we construct the history of ideas is Michel Foucault. For Foucault neither the etic or the emic exist outside of the power structures of the prevailing discourse (Foucault 1972). Because Foucault approaches both system and life-world views in this way he undermines not just modernist reason but also the privileged or centred subject (Scheurich and Bell McKenzie 2005: 848). That is, he is undermining human agency, our capacity to act in ways that shape our lives. This analytic view presents a challenge to the practical project in this book. The challenge we have set ourselves is to identify ways we can legitimize insider views so they can shape what is considered appropriate in prevailing understandings of need and in assessments of how to meet that need. That is, to colonize the etic by the insights of the emic. But Foucault is arguing that neither are free from the constraints of the prevailing discourse. We will revisit this argument throughout the book and will keep our confidence in the benefits of accessing and acting upon the subjective. We think there are places in Foucault's work where even he is more amenable to such an approach: we also return to this.

Our life-world/emic contributions in this chapter come from the personal accounts of relatives and staff and fictional depictions of care for people with dementia. We will insert their contribution into our predominantly system world/etic presentation and will ask in our final sections of this chapter what these accounts bring to the assessment of quality of care and quality of life for those living and dying with dementia and what they add to our understanding about the space there is for effecting change.

The rise of quality

Where 'quality' comes from

Across health and social care provision, and particularly marked where the focus is on care rather than cure, there has been an elevation of the importance of quality as a construct which is used both to define the objective of an intervention and as a measure of its outcome. Indeed, quality has become an ubiquitous concept, often unchallenged, an assumed 'hurrah' word. Surely people must all be in favour of quality (Harrison and Mort 1998)? However, there is no consensus about the meaning of quality: 'it is put to different uses to serve different purposes and its meaning changes accordingly' (Pfeffer and Coote 1991: i). Many of the ideas about quality in health and social care have emanated from the world of manufacturing and business. Alaszewski and Manthorpe (1993) argue that quality is 'associated with the development of post-Fordist management in the private sector, and the transfer of these concepts to the public sector as part of a new public management' (1993: 653–4). A Fordist model is concerned to deliver maximum quantity at lowest cost, the car assembly line at Ford being the personification of such an approach. When transferred to the welfare state, Fordist approaches saw services developed in ways that were determined by those providing them, rather than being determined by those for whom they were meant. As a consequence, standard products were supplied irrespective of need. People using services would be required to fit in to the prevailing practice. (Henry Ford said about his Model T Ford car, 'You can have any colour you like as long as it is black'.) Hospitals were built in standard sizes and with standard layout: they did not always reflect geographic patterns of need and they appeared to be staffed and run in ways that served the institution, for example, with respect to visiting times and meal times. The NHS was product-oriented rather than consumer-oriented (Harrison et al. 1989).

It was the arrival of a market orientation into welfare provision that precipitated a change in this Fordist model. This followed a shift in the prevailing ethos of manufacturing. The market in consumer durables had become saturated and there was no longer a simple rationale for firms to maximize output and minimize cost. In a post-Fordist world private sector organizations began to emphasize the importance of getting the product right and prioritizing quality.

These changes in the way priorities were set in manufacturing are important for our argument because in the UK, and elsewhere in the world, there was an attempt to replicate the changing ideology of business within health and social care provision. This might appear counterintuitive, as providing care is not like producing automobiles and, in the UK, manufacturing was in decline as a sector of the economy. Seeking to replicate its approaches appeared perverse. However, a series of central government policy initiatives have taken business approaches and sought to integrate them into mainstream health and social care provision.

In 1989, the publication of the *Working for Patients* White Paper (Department of Health 1989) developed what was now being called a 'market approach' by allowing and encouraging an internal market in health, whereby some NHS staff, primarily GPs, became purchasers and some, primarily hospitals, providers of health care (Small 1989). The expectation was that market forces would improve efficiency and quality (Enthovan 1985). By the mid-1990s, it was not unusual to have private sector companies advising the NHS, assuming a similarity between their wish to sell more groceries, for example, and the optimizing of health care delivery. A divisional director of Marks and Spencer (a leading UK retail chain) told an NHS conference that 'although the definition of "patient" and "customer" were quite different', both Marks and Spencer and the NHS were involved in providing solutions to people's needs. 'We both offer a service to the public and we both need to be concerned with quality and value for money' (Giles 1993: 15). The level of banality captured in such statements did not seem to prevent their widespread dissemination of such a view into the culture of health care.

This approach lasted until the innovations of a new Labour administration and the restructuring of the NHS consequent upon the White Paper, *The new NHS: modern dependable* in 1997 (Department of Health 1997). As well as abolishing the internal market this introduced new sets of national standards and mechanisms to examine them – National Service Frameworks, National Institute of Clinical Effectiveness, National Performance Assessment Framework. There would be a National Survey of Patient and User Experience to monitor adherence to standards. Performance Assessment and Clinical Governance would ensure that quality standards were maintained. At the same time the reforms shifted responsibility for commissioning services to local primary care organizations.

A further reorganization, in the summer of 2005, *Commissioning a patient-led NHS*, focuses on commissioning from primary care organizations, which have been drastically reduced in number (Department of Health 2005). This was followed by another White Paper, *Our health, our care, our say* (Department of Health 2006a) which sought to provide a more integrated and more locally based and responsive health and social care service. In November 2006 another new initiative, the Dignity in Care campaign, was launched to seek to ensure older people were treated with dignity in hospital and in care homes. They were to be delivered services in a 'person-centred way'. (www.dh.gov.uk/PolicyAnd-Guidance/HealthandSocialCareTopics/SocialCare/ accessed 20 December 2006).

Hence, there is a history of concerns with how to produce optimal quality services that has seen three stages. First, it was assumed that the best quality was what the professionals decided was needed. This reflects a paternalism that was widespread in all areas of health and social care and that has far from disappeared. Secondly, the focus shifted to the idea that if people had a choice standards would be driven up because the better services would thrive and the weaker services would either have to adapt to the standards of the better or be replaced. Third, there is the idea that there should be top-down standard-setting and local involvement, including contacts with service users, to ensure local needs are recognized.

There is now a wide proliferation of assumptions underlying different approaches to quality. There is not just one understanding: if a person proposes that quality should be maximized as a goal of care then one should ask 'what is quality?' How this is answered shapes who is involved, the end points aspired to and the measures used to identify success, as illustrated in Table 5.1.

There are also 'whole system' approaches which do not rely just on expert knowledge and professional definitions, for example the Pursuing Perfection programme. Its components include a concern with patients and users as partners in decision-making in their own care, with targets and multidimensional measurement of performance (Kabcenell and Roessner 2002). The principle at the heart of Pursuing Perfection then is that the patient defines quality and that definition is cascaded down through the small units of care, the micro-system which they are directly involved with, the organization that supports that micro-system and the external environment that shapes the behaviour of that organization. The quality of all the levels is determined by their impact on the patient.

Not in favour of quality?

There are critical voices, both with a pragmatic and systemic perspective, arguing that a focus on quality is not helpful. Pragmatic voices question how

Table 5.1 Different ways of thinking about quality[1] (see Pfeffer and Coote 1991)

Model	Key characteristics	Key outcome
Traditional	A service that is superior to others – one with prestige and relative advantage over others	Improved quality of environment equates with better service
Scientific/expert	The organization is 'fit for purpose' – quality is its ability to meet a specific need	A series of measures of activity and outcome including: clinical audit; accreditation by external organizations; standard setting
Excellence	The total quality management model. Meet 'customers' requirements	Organizing and involving the whole organization, every department, every activity, every single person at every level
Consumerist	Empower consumers	Growth of organization promoting consumer power – or charters to formalize standards (Cantley et al. 2005; Age Concern 2002)

[1] We are grateful to Kevin Mitchell for his guidance in identifying quality models

far progress can be made in the UK public sector given entrenched professional identities, change-fatigued staff, badly designed and distributed facilities, shortcomings in training and in supervisory skills in relation to the different ways of working a focus on quality would involve. The list of major reforms in the NHS, in a period of a relatively few years, would suggest that there is not long enough to build in, audit and enhance quality initiatives before another reorganization arrives. Perhaps there is a paradox between reforms ostensibly to improve care and the time needed to make the systemic, attitudinal and training changes required to make sure quality improves at all levels in the organization and particularly at the level of patient care.

There are also more systemic criticisms of quality. How can it be measured? How can the different perceptions of quality be reconciled? How does pursuing quality fit with other policy imperatives – for example evidence-based practice? More fundamentally, 'is quality good for you?' (Pfeffer and Coote 1991). It is intrinsically problematic to prioritize quality in welfare organizations because the organization's aims are invariably multifaceted. Since any individual's perception of quality is likely to vary across time, just as his or her circumstances change, how can the service be flexible enough to meet these changing needs? It is likely that a person will experience a variety of different contexts of care and what is seen as being of high quality may be different in each. We may define quality differently in terms of the care delivered by, for example, a consultant neurologist or by a carer helping with personal hygiene. Welfare also has a counter imperative that is concerned with equality, which is not necessarily reconcilable with quality if quality is understood as just meeting an individual's present needs. Does a concern with quality also inhibit risk-taking? The emergence of new forms of care that may be better than the homogenous 'high quality' ones that stay close to the familiar, may be impeded because of the risk of straying into unfamiliar territory. An important concern to reduce risk, often in the name of ensuring patient safety, may be bad for quality in that enhancing quality may require risk-taking.

Is quality misunderstood as a scientific or norm-based aspiration when in reality it is better understood as pertaining to an aesthetic understanding of what is life-enhancing for a person? Quality is not reducible to something captured in a concept like fitness for purpose, a criterion that might be appropriate if for example, a washing machine were being discussed. Finally, is quality just used rhetorically, for example to divert discussion about absolute levels of support and/or the distribution of support? Is it part of 'the never ending search for, and fascination with technical solutions to political problems' (Hunter 1993: 29).

A concern with quality may also divert us from a more commonplace, but perhaps even more difficult thing to achieve, that is to engage with people with respect. In Michael Ignatieff's novel *Scar Tissue* (1993) the narrator is talking to his mother's doctor about how he would like his mother to be interacted with. His mother has dementia. The narrator says:

> 'A lot depends on whether people like you treat her as a human being or not. She needs respect. Just giving her the benefit of the doubt. Just assuming there might be some method in her madness. Not humouring her – but acting as if she is rational, as if she knows what she is saying.'.
>
> The doctor replies saying, 'Isn't that just humouring her?'

> (Ignatieff 1993: 59)

The narrator also considers why staff can differ so much:

> Some nurses seemed possessed of an intuitive natural tenderness towards their patients while others did not ... others, not necessarily less decent people, who had to have procedures to behave decently, who had no natural intuition for what would insult the honour of strangers.

> (Ignatieff 1993: 110)

Working with differing approaches to quality

Debates about quality matter because they shape the system imperatives within which services are planned and delivered. Specifically, for those with dementia who are dying and have end of life care needs, a number of problems are raised in relation to system imperatives and the quality of care:

- Fordism sees quality standards set by providers of goods and services. This leads to a lack of sensitivity to the needs of people being cared for. It is a characteristic evident in care of older people where it has been seen in the past in the establishment of large, impersonal, hospitals that have been characterized as akin to 'factory facilities', or 'human warehouses' (Sheldon 1961) .

- A market orientation can result in the proliferation of providers in the end of life care field, some within and some outside state provision, some for profit and some not-for-profit. These can be found in the form of hospitals, home care teams, day care: hospices, and long-term care settings such as nursing homes and care homes. The problem is their distribution and availability. There is variability both geographically and according to diagnosis and there is considerable variation in the standards of care they offer. There is not a clear sense of what purchasers of care should be insisting upon. This approach equates choice with quality – i.e. if you can choose then quality will be encouraged as providers seek to remain in the 'market'. But choice does not only do this. Choice also leads to providers competing on ground as close to their 'competitors' as possible, but seeking to do so with slightly lower costs. If your needs are for a different sort of residential care the idea of market choice does not mean you will find it – you may just find lots of similar places, none of which meet your needs. (The soft drinks market provides an analogy – you can 'choose' between Pepsi and Coca-Cola.) There is also a problematic absence of choice in the sense that one cannot choose not to access care. There is not a 'no purchase option' (you can choose to have neither Pepsi or Coca-Cola!)

- Standard-setting and local involvement, a top-down and bottom-up approach, would seem to offer more possibilities for the development of effective and appropriate services. The characteristic pattern of service use in dementia is one that sees a person moving in and out of a number of different care settings, with a need to not only offer care within each setting but handle the changes between them. Hence the recognition of whole system understandings of quality and the value of comparison and 'benchmarking' to set standards. The 'involvement' approach to quality characteristically relies on two options for service users. The first is 'exit' – choosing not to stay in, or with, a service if it is not seen to be of satisfactory quality. The second is 'voice', that is the opportunity to express one's dissatisfaction and to have that expression listened to. Both these areas are problematic for end of life care and for dementia care.

Much of the push to build 'quality' in health and social care comes from top-down regimes of standard-setting, inspection and the imposition of financial penalties and the presence of incentives. This can ameliorate or eradicate inherent structural problems such as the number, qualification and skill-mix of staff at a centre, the nature of the physical environment, the acceptable protocols for admission, transfer, discharge; and it can address care practices – the use of restraints or of psychotropic medicine, for example. Legislating and enforcing minimum acceptable standards below which no care setting should fall has considerable importance given a history of geriatric, dementia and end of life care where there have been many examples of services falling below these minimum standards. As we observed in Chapter 3, a major spur to the development of hospices was the observations made, and studies done over the last 50 years, into the inadequacy of provision for older people and specifically for the chronically sick and for dying individuals.

Despite legislative changes and successful initiatives in some areas of care of older people, contemporary studies in many parts of the world repeat the concerns of 50 years of critical studies when they invoke and repeat descriptions of care facilities as being like human 'warehouses' and explanations for the relative neglect of older ill people such as 'out of sight out of mind' (Godlove *et al.* 2004). That such descriptions are regularly and repeatedly invoked is resonant of the intractability of the problems besetting the care of the elderly and chronically sick. Ballard *et al.* (2001a), in a small survey in 2001, identified no care homes offering even a fair standard of care.

As well as the regulatory framework addressing some of the structural shortcomings of care there are considerable challenges in how care is delivered, even within a regulated environment. It is widely observed that in care homes one encounters the paradox that members of our society with many of the most complex needs are being looked after by people with the least training, supervision, job security and with pay at or near the statutory minimum. In practice, the nature of care environments in the areas we are focusing on means that it is the quality of personal interactions that is key (see Kitwood 1997a), something for which it is not easy to regulate. Writing about the USA, but of widespread relevance, Applebaum sums up what is a perverse state of affairs:

> In most communities teenagers working in fast food establishments earn more than home care, assisted living, or nursing home workers ... nursing homes are second only to nuclear power in their regulatory requirements ... [1] yet few would argue that any sector of long- term care is well regulated.
>
> (Applebaum 2001: ix)

---

[1] This is an example of the 'inverse care law' (Tudor-Hart 1971: 412). This captures a tendency for areas with the least intense need to have the best health services, or at least the most resources, and conversely the areas with most need having the least.

In our summary of the emergence of the quality agenda we identified the dependence on the importance of the idea of markets and choice as the means to drive up standards. A number of commentators have noted that there is a conflict between top-down standard setting and the idea of local choice. Perri 6 and Peck (2004) argue that in the UK the New Labour project in public services creates a 'hybrid between hierarchy and individualism'. Broad policy initiatives are characterized both by a need to regulate and a wish to shift accountability away from central government. The hierarchical component is defined via a series of standards and inspection, often reinforced via financial incentives or penalties. Individualism becomes possible because there are spaces even within a highly governed environment where it is possible to take initiatives and through this to 'earn autonomy' (Perri 6 and Peck 2004: 101). Examples exist in both the world of palliative care and dementia care in which innovators have explored spaces left in systems to pursue local innovations and through these offer alternative models of what services can do. One is reminded of Dame Cicely Saunders' decision to set up St Christopher's Hospice outside the NHS – so that the ideas it generated would be able to move back in (Clark 1999). The sorts of autonomy we are considering here, and the innovations that follow, are system world (etic) concerns. When the life-world is looked to it cannot be just assumed that because something is innovatory it will be welcomed by patients, or that it will resonate with emic concerns.

The crucial question here is to consider how far quality of care, as understood in the system world of policy-makers and health professionals, captures the life-world assumptions of patients and carers. That is to consider the challenge that the word *and* creates in a desire to improve system and life-world quality. Consider two different ways of approaching the question of what is important in the care people receive:

1. Is the way care is delivered the most important variable? Ignatieff distinguishes between necessary and sufficient requirements to ensure the dignity and respect of others. It is necessary to provide income support and medical care but it is not sufficient. The manner of giving support, and its moral basis, determines the experience:

   > whether strangers at my door get their stories listened to by the social worker, whether the ambulance man takes care not to jostle them when they are taken down the steep stairs of their apartment building, whether a nurse sits with them in the hospital when they are frightened and alone. Respect and dignity are conferred by gestures such as these. They are gestures too much a matter of human art to be made a consistent matter of administrative routine.

   (Ignatieff 1984: 16)

2. Alternatively, could it be that the most important factor is not how things are provided but how effective they are? That is, it is not process but outcome that is paramount. Aneurin Bevan's statement, 'I would rather be kept alive in the efficient if cold altruism of a large hospital than expire in a gush of warm sympathy in a small one' (see Klein 1989: 75–6) sums up this position. One may easily counter his point by arguing that it is problematic when the intention is not cure, but it should not assumed that because people have been classified as having illnesses where 'the treatment intention is not cure' they have forsaken the socially resilient belief in the miraculous power of science to make an exception for them. In the years when large numbers in the UK were dying with AIDS there were reports by doctors that knowledgeable patients would still wait for their doctor to return from a scientific conference with the cure (for them) in their briefcase (Small 1993). Both the emic and etic can harbour miraculous wishes and magical thinking – it is just that the idea of what is magic will differ between that held by, say, the doctor and the patient.

The difference between necessary and sufficient requirements of care are vividly contrasted in Margaret Forster's (1989) novel, *Have the Men Had Enough?* Her character, Jenny, is thinking about the care of her mother-in-law who has dementia and reflecting on her visit to a 'highly recommended home':

> I cannot wait to see again some of these people who raved about the Green Valley Home. They are either blind or deaf or wilfully wicked. Did they not see the six beds in a room, all jammed together? The lack of pictures, of any decorations, anything personal? Did they not see, at eleven o'clock in the morning, the twenty chairs in a circle in a silent, dark room, each with a motionless figure slumped on it? Did they count the lavatories, only two of them, both up flights of stairs? Did they not smell the urine, certainly not masked by disinfectant? Did they not hear the silence, the lack of activity? Did they not sense the utter despair? Maybe they did and told themselves, it did not matter because Grandma or Granddad was past it, it did not matter because everything was the same to them. As long as it is clean (it was) and warm (it was) and the staff are kind (they appeared to be) then *that* was what mattered.

(Forster 1989: 61)

Quality of care

The messiness of subjectivities

So far in this chapter, the focus has been a general one. We have considered conceptualizations of quality and the historical evolution and social policy significance of these. We have related these ways of addressing quality to the concerns of dementia and palliative care. We now turn to a more specific description of how ways to maximize quality of care have been operationalized. We will then go on to examine understandings of quality of life.

Our discussion about the rise of quality has led us to the position of identifying how quality of care can be approached via one of two epistemologies. The first is a positivist one in which judgements are made about structures, inputs and processes and in which measurement, standards and inspection in particular settings of care are utilized (the system world). In the second, quality of care is subjective and is about the experience (the life-world) of the recipient of a service. Our specific focus on end of life care has underlined the importance of the subjective. But our argument also has to recognize the power located in the system world. Hence, we have to consider how to access the subjective and how to communicate its significance in such a way that it does not appear alien to the system world and to the guardians of an epistemology of measurement within it. We have to do this without compromising the subjective's nuanced and contingent nature. An example might be if we distinguish between the quality of care and the quality of caring, a distinction flagged by Ignatieff's distinction between necessary and sufficient responses to ensure care is given in a way that recognizes the dignity of its givers and recipients, referred to above. Quality of care commonly is used to structure discussions about the number and skill-mix of staff, about how far procedures accord with best practice guidelines and so on. Quality of caring, in contrast, refers to the humanity and respect with which that care is provided (Glass 1991).

Of course, what we can access subjectively may reveal that things are happening in the system world, or in the subjectivity of other people's life-world, which are very different from our own experience. Forster's fictional Jenny, daughter-in-law of the woman she calls 'Grandma' and who has dementia, has an encounter with a different world view on the day Grandma moves into a new care home:

> Then the minute we were inside, we were confronted by an old woman on a walking frame coming towards us, inching her way painfully along the corridor. Grandma began tut-tutting and poor-souling and I wished we could avoid a confrontation. But we could not. The old woman pushed her walking-frame right up to us and said to Grandma 'They put you in here to die – don't you believe anything they tell you – that's what they do, put us here to die'.

> (Forster 1989: 179)

Grandma then has a fall and is admitted to a long-stay psychogeriatric ward. Now Jenny sees that it is not just the staff, or the setting, that shapes the sort of place you are in, but it is also the others you are sharing it with:

> On the way we passed a row of six chairs. Upon each was what looked like a dead occupant. One was twisted into a grotesque attitude, head back at an unnatural angle,

feet splayed out, arms flung wide. One was bowed over. Head almost touching the toes. The others had their eyes open but did not blink or move.

(Forster 1989: 202)

Embracing subjectivity leaves you in a messy place, because it leaves you interacting with the subjectivity of others.

Frameworks for assessing quality of care

Quality of care is assessed via a wide range of indicators (Chassin *et al.* 1998). Many of them draw on Donabedien's framework which directs attention to structure, process and outcome. Initial work utilizing this approach focused disproportionately on structure, details of the physical attributes of the place of care and the levels and qualification of staff most notably (Donabedien 1980, 1988). Process concerns have subsequently emerged as a focus of concern. They have most typically included a consideration of what is done (appropriateness), when it is done (timeliness) and how well it is done (technical proficiency). An important dimension that augments the Donabedien framework underlines the appreciation that it is the overall experience of care, the care pathway, that should be the focus, not just one institution. People most typically move from place to place as their condition and circumstances change (Noelker and Harel 2001: 7).

There has been a proliferation of problem specific guidelines and standards designed to assess quality of care in long-term care, chronic illness and end of life care. Typically they have a line of reporting back to professionals in funding, commissioning or regulatory agencies. They are often, in essence, modifications of tools developed in acute care settings, even though acute care characteristically has a different ethos of care. Problems in theorizing the philosophical assumptions of long-term care and problems in identifying what would be acceptable outcomes in chronic illness and end of life care mean that it is no surprise when it is concluded that, despite the sophisticated tools and measurement procedures the concept of quality and its relationship to organizational characteristics remains unclear (Sainfort *et al.* 1995). Not least is the challenge, also broached in palliative care, that the outcome of most significance is quality of life and that quality of life constitutes a category difference from the structures, processes and outcomes that contribute to usual conceptualizations of quality of care. Quality of life, in this reading, cannot be identified via technical measures and according to professionally defined ideals.

Audit

While there has been a long history of concern with the standards of care provided, and while there have been links made between this and individual and organizational competence (Rosser 1985), it is only relatively recently that this concern has been generalized such that it is a system world aspiration that all care providers, and all care provided, will be audited to see that the best possible standards are being achieved. Further, if it is not, then it is assumed that ameliorative (or disciplinary) interventions will be instigated, and correspondingly that if best standards are being met then there will be rewards – prestige, financial benefits, the opportunity to expand. These are changes that are manifest in the rise in prominence of audit, indeed in the ascendancy of an audit culture.

Audit is a cyclical process that can focus on both clinical care and organizational performance. Audit would have us:

◆ Observe practice to see how far it is achieving goals set against an agreed standard or benchmark;

◆ Modify practice to help what is provided approach more closely to the levels aimed for;

◆ Begin the process again, ideally now pursuing higher standards.

See Box 5.1 for two examples.

Box 5.1 Examples of audit in palliative care

Organizational:
Cancer Relief Macmillan Fund (1994). The aim is to identify overall activity via assessing practice according to 11 standards. These include: service values; management structures, team work, physical environment, staff development and support. Assessors consider how far each standard is being met and recommend improvements. Standards of particular relevance for this chapter include ones that examine how far the care environment is conducive to independence and participation by patients, and ones that requires patients and family needs to be assessed, planned, implemented and evaluated on an individual basis.

Clinical:
Support Team Assessment Schedule (STAS) (Higginson and McCarthy 1993). A 17-item schedule to assess outcomes, intermediate outcomes and outputs, including pain and symptom control, anxiety, communication. Relies on the assessment of professionals.

Quality of care in palliative care

The conventional way of identifying the goals of palliative care is to categorize them as follows:

+ pain and symptom control
+ improving the patient's quality of life
+ relieving fears and anxieties
+ care for family members/carers.

There follows the possibility that approaches can be devised and implemented to measure how effective a particular care setting, or particular carers, are in achieving these goals both for individual patients and for all those they care for. If one then expands the remit of what palliative care is seeking to do – for example, to addressing spiritual needs – then further means of assessing the impact of a service can be added (Higginson 1998). More recent conceptualizations which set goals related to health-promoting palliative care or to the potential of palliative care to contribute to healthy cities (Kellehear 2005) set new challenges in devising audit measures to assess achievement against aspiration, or against potential achievement – do you measure activity against what you say you will do or what a reasonable person would calculate you should be able to do given your resources and context? We return to the wider health-promoting possibilities of palliative care in Chapter 7.

Quality of care in dementia care

One way of assessing quality of care in palliative care is to ask patients about it, usually via interviews and/or questionnaires. In dementia care this remains a possible route at early and mid stages and later in the illness if one is prepared to embrace a wider repertoire of communicative practice. One part of that repertoire involves using structured observations of behaviour and affect (see Brooker 1995). Observational methods characteristically study and seek to quantify type and level of activity, including the quality of activity and interaction. Examples include the Quality of Interactions Schedule (Dean *et al.* 1993) and Dementia Care Mapping (DCM) (Kitwood and Bredin 1993). We will expand, by way of example, on DCM.

DCM starts from the assumption that for people with dementia well-being is a direct result of the quality of relationships they enjoy with those around them. Devising DCM was 'a serious attempt to take the standpoint of the person with dementia, using a combination of empathy and observational skill' (Kitwood 1997a: 4). It is, essentially, a means of recording interaction and lack of interaction and then using the results with staff to seek to improve their

Table 5.2 Constituent parts of the DCM observational tool

	Focus	Measure
Quality of life	Relative well-being Affect	Behavioural category code – 24 different domains of behaviour – further qualified according to their impact on well-being
	Engagement Occupation	Relative state of well-being or ill-being in a fixed time period (WIB score)
Quality of care	Impact of staff behaviour on personhood	Personal detractions – staff behaviour that has the potential to undermine personhood, coded by type and severity Personal enhancers – those behaviours that enhance personhood

practice. Its aim is 'to systematically move dementia care from primarily a custodial and task-focused model into one that respects people with dementia as human beings' (Brooker 2005: 12).

As is illustrated in Table 5.2, DCM is structured around a focus on both quality of life and quality of care. There have been some attempts to ascertain concurrent validity of DCM scores, specifically that part of the quality of life sections of DCM that address relative well-being or ill-being in a fixed time period (known as the WIB score) and staff proxy quality of life measures (Edelman *et al.* 2004). Overall, some moderately significant correlations, in specific sorts of settings and specific sorts of people, have been identified.

There has been progress in developing DCM in a dynamic way such that it can link observation, training and practice improvement, verified via further observation (scrutiny and oversight). Of particular significance for us is DCM's identification that a necessary prerequisite for understanding quality requires changes to be assessed against their contribution to enhancing the self. It can be argued that the extent to which the self is enhanced can only be assessed with the involvement of those receiving care and members of their informal support system.

Quality of life

Contemplating what quality of life is and how it can be enhanced, or how it is under attack, has a high profile in popular discourse. It is also increasingly evident in relation to employment practice, where the work–life balance is now considered a relevant subject for employers to engage with and in health policy where a concern with quality of life and with the linked concept of well-being is being given increasing prominence. In what follows we are going to examine understandings about quality of life as they apply to ill people and in particular to people with illnesses where there is no cure. In popular discussion there is an assumption that if quality of life is addressed it is about seeking improvements. As such a concern with quality of life is consistent with the modernist conceit that the natural direction of our life and our times is that things should improve, and that it is within our control to bring our reason and science to bear to achieve this improvement. When illnesses without cure are considered the concern is often deterioration in quality of life, and the focus is on preservation of quality of life or amelioration of the effects of any deterioration. Those living with illnesses that cannot be cured are cast out of the embrace of modernity into a pre, or postmodern world. These are spaces characterized by fate and faith or by contingency, and we will explore them in more detail in Chapter 6.

A focus on illness and quality of life is ethically problematic in that it allows for the possibility that situations may be contemplated where the quality of a life is so bad that a life has no value (See Jennings 2004). Box 5.2 examines the relationship between quality of life and ethics and Box 5.3 provides a reminder,

Box 5.2 Quality of life and ethics

(a) Ways that use of the term quality of life can detract from ethics (from Jennings 2004)

Cohen (1983) argues that using a term like quality of life suggests that life is not intrinsically worthy of respect, that is, it can have greater or lesser value according to circumstances. A danger with engaging in discussions about quality of life is the flawed reasoning that can come next – 'the idea of quality of life necessarily turns into a judgement about the value of human life. (This mistaken line of reasoning goes something like this: "A life of very poor quality is not worth living. If a life is not worth living, then it had no value")' (Jennings 2004: 268).

(b) Ways that use of the term quality of life can enhance ethics:

It is essential to distinguish quality of life from value or worth of life.

Quality of life can be used to enhance respect for all as part of one moral community.

Quality of life can be used to support calls for social reform and better services, making a case on social justice and equity lines.

Box 5.3 Who defines what is quality of life?

March 2006, UK. Baby MB – 19 months old with genetic condition, spinal muscular atrophy, which leads to almost total paralysis. Doctors argued before the court that 'his quality of life was so poor that he should be allowed to die'. MB's parents argued that he was conscious, could probably see, hear and feel and take pleasure from, for example, contact with his family. 'It's what is going on inside and not what's on the outside', argued MB's mother. The doctors felt that treatment to prolong life caused suffering and did harm. But was the baby suffering intolerably? His parents said no. One problem is that the child cannot be asked directly and that there is no measure to say what is 'intolerable'.

through a consideration of the disagreements over Baby MB, that what constitutes quality of life depends on the position from which that life is viewed. These are important issues with which to engage given the social death and denial of personhood that has been characteristic of much of the experience of those nearing death and of those with dementia, and given a continuing presence of a euthanasia lobby. Proposing the value of quality of life measures may, thus, constitute something of a wolf in sheep's clothing, using an understandable assumption that a focus on quality is benign, indeed enlightened, to argue that some lives have no quality and if this is the case then it is justifiable to hasten their end.

Philosophically, a concern with quality of life has more often been captured within a consideration as to what constitutes a good life. This has been a perennial part of philosophy, for example Aristotle's *Ethics* is concerned with examining what constitutes 'the good'. The study of the good life, in the post Enlightenment West, has been dominated by just one theory – individualism. This argues that no one but the 'owner' of a life is in a position to say if it is a good life. The accompanying ethical principle is one of autonomy which is elevated to a pre-eminent, (and often unquestioned) position. We have returned at many points in this book to the challenges of prevalent assumptions such as the assumption of the ethical importance of autonomy on end of life care and dementia care (see chapter four). Limitations on the pre-eminence of individualism and autonomy are few. Children are seen as 'not yet autonomous'. The assumption is that there is some objective good that parents pursue on behalf of the child. The scope of this may diminish as the child's capacity increases.

We might also contemplate a category of the 'no longer autonomous' that a person with terminal illness, and particularly a person with dementia, could be assigned to with the possibility of a pre-category of 'becoming less autonomous' – a time when some areas of independent action are denied to them. (See Hockey and James 1993 on a distinction between growing up and growing old.)

One of the problems with individualism and autonomy is that it can appear that some people are favoured. In his book *Untold Stories* Alan Bennett describes Hilda, who is a resident of the same nursing home as his mother. Like his mother, Hilda has dementia. But Hilda refuses to eat at mealtimes, and a combination of this and the staff's busyness and lack of attention to her eating and drinking, means she is starving.

> Demented or not, if Hilda were a child there would be a story to tell and blame attaching. But Hilda is at the end of her life not the beginning. Even so, were she a Nobel Prize winner, or not a widow from Darwen but the last survivor of Bloomsbury, yes, then an effort might be made. As it is she is gradually slipping away, which is what this place is for. The water creeps over the sand.

> (Bennett 2005: 116)

Individualism and autonomy are pre-eminent assumptions in the prevailing understanding about what the prerequisites of quality of life are, but they do not define what quality of life consists of. There are different ways of approaching the idea of what are the components of quality of life.

1. Sensation (hedonic) theories – happiness and pleasure are constituents of good quality of life, pain and unhappiness define a poor quality of life.

2. Reasonable preference theories – satisfaction of a person's rational desires or preferences are what is necessary for good quality of life.

3. Theories of human flourishing – to the extent that an individual continues to grow and flourish their quality of life is enhanced.

4. Salutogenic theory – this argues that there is a link between one's sense of coherence and of the comprehensibility, manageability and meaningfulness of life and that it is this link that underpins quality. This sense of coherence can emanate from a spiritual dimension (see Antonovsky 1979, 1987; McCubbin *et al.* 1998).

There are also other ways of thinking about quality of life that do not locate its achievement entirely within the self:

1. Reintegration to normal living can be seen as a proxy for quality of life, via what is a rehabilitative ethic (Schag and Heinrich 1990). This can include a focus on what a person can still do rather than what they can no longer do (see Kleinman 1988).

2. A community-centred understanding is based on a consideration of quality of life that looks at the individual as he or she interacts with those around them, both in immediate circles of care and in the wider networks touched by their illness (Ware 1984).

Quality of life can also be approached via a moral perspective (see Jennings 2004). Hence, quality of life can be considered:

1. As a property of the individual. Quality of life is not fixed, it can be changed by your own or others' actions. There is no straightforward moral significance in the level of quality identified. That is, a poor quality of life is not a sign of moral failing.

2. As a goal of care. The moral point of our dealings with another is to sustain and improve quality of life. The onus here is on the care giver not receiver – the former can be judged by what they achieve, the latter can not.

3. As part of a person's being in the world. Quality of life resides in the interaction between a person and their social and physical environment.

4. As a measure of the gap between the *actual* circumstances and the *possible* circumstances of an intrinsically valuable life (Jennings 2004: 270).

Is quality best understood as a comparison or an absolute? Should one group be compared with another, one person with another, the past with the present, or should comparisons be made between what happens with the best that could happen? Alternatively, should quality be approached as a concept that can identify different states without the need to rank these states on a continuum of good to bad? Perhaps quality is forever shifting. Perhaps at an instant it captures many different things.

We do not wish to labour the esoteric world of the quality of life gurus. For our more limited purpose we want to highlight that all of the approaches in the lists above present problems for people living and dying with dementia. Assumptions about pain and unhappiness, absence of rationality, no possibility of flourishing, and an absence of meaningfulness; no thoughts on reintegration, strained circles of care and a sense that there are no positives that could provide a counterweight to the illness are all evident in responses to dementia. Further, such assumptions suggest that people with dementia can readily be disenfranchised in a system world that makes decisions based on assessments of quality. As we argued at the start of this section there is also the danger that a focus on quality, and the identification of its absence, can lead to an assumption that some lives have no value because they have no/low quality.

Many different ways of understanding quality can be seen in palliative care and, to an extent, in dementia care. However, in dementia the notion of quality of life as the property of an individual has been dominant. As Jennings has argued, an assumption that you need to know you are happy to be happy 'will load the dice against Alzheimer's disease' (Jennings 2004: 5). This individual approach has dominated to the detriment of the recognition that responsibility can lie in the caregiver and that with dementia there is a difference between the actual and the possible. This gap between the actual and possible has not always been recognized in the milieu of therapeutic pessimism that has pervaded much provision, a gap that could be addressed with a focus on seeing quality as located in the social and physical environment.

Dementia poses a particular challenge to prevailing conceptualizations of quality of life. As such it has proved rich ground for meditations as to alternative understandings that do not shy away from engaging with both the conceptual and the practical challenges (see Bond 1999; Post 2000b: Jennings 2000; Hughes 2005).

Measuring quality of life

We now shift from debates that focus on conceptualizing quality of life to those where the emphasis is on how to measure it.

Functionalists and phenomenologists

If one adopts a functionalist approach to quality of life measurement then aspects of a person's life can be identified and measured. For example, scales to record the performance of the activities of everyday living: personal care, domestic roles, mobility, and to record how far an individual can carry out social roles in relation to work, finance, and family life can be devised. The scales seek to identify how far a particular illness impacts on one's abilities in these areas. These are nomothetic approaches – they seek to measure traits based on preconceived assumptions as to the components of quality of life.

In contrast, there is a phenomenological, or hermeneutic approach (an idiographic way of approaching quality of life). Here, the assumption is that one constructs an understanding of quality of life through the identification of those things unique to individuals. These can then be considered in so far as they impact on each other, at specific times, and on how far they interact to generate an overall sense of quality of life (see Bowling 1997: 37–9). Bowling (1995) illustrated the potential gap between the nomothetic and idiographic when she compared answers to a national population survey with answers to open-ended qualitative questions seeking to identify, 'what were the most important areas of one's life, and what were the most important areas of life affected by your illness'? There were differences in each set of answers and the answers to the illness questions included areas not included in precoded questions.

Following a functionalist/phenomenologist distinction, quality of life measures adopt one of two main approaches (Box 5.4). The first presents a person with a series of constructs and questions, each with a range of answers, usually identifying degrees of experience, e.g. from no pain to unbearable pain. From these answers a composite picture is built up. It essentially relies on psychometric testing. This is an approach that has become ever more sophisticated. For example, the European Organizations for Research and Treatment of Cancer (EORTC) quality of life scale combines a core tool with disease-specific add-ons (Aaronson *et al.* 1988). It is also possible to give different

Box 5.4 Examples of approaching functionalist measures from different starting points

Quality of life is in inverse relationship between an individuals' expectations and the reality of their situation (Calman's gap) (Calman 1984).

Most quality of life questionnaires implicitly operate on this system, i.e. an individual ranks themself not according to some absolute but according to what, for them, is normal. A change in quality of life can occur if either condition or expectation changes.

Utility concept – compare present with normal functioning

For example, one may give normal functioning a value of 1 and death a value of 0. Present functioning is assessed along this continuum and this allows a comparison over time. For example, are you worse after a specific intervention than before it (Clinch *et al.* 1998: 83).

(i) Q-TWiST (time without symptoms and toxicity) (Gelber *et al.* 1993) – this provides a way for assigning a lower assessment of quality to time with symptoms and to time with toxicity caused by treatment.

(ii) Time trade-off – McNeil *et al.* (1981) explored treatment options in laryngeal cancer – would people choose possibly longer survival with loss of speech or shorter survival while retaining speech (the choice involved surgery or radiation treatment)? What one chose in this study related to the work the person asked did. For example, executives chose speech more than firefighters. This sort of approach can be adapted for chronic pain, would you choose complete analgesia regardless of sedation (Clinch *et al.* 1998: 84) i.e. trade-off pain against wakefulness? Others options could be approached in this way also.

weight to subscales. Hence, one could score very highly in terms of overall quality of life even if one was experiencing high levels of pain. That such a situation is frequently encountered in clinical care is illustrative of the danger of simple attributional systems that assume if one is near to death then one's quality of life or even one's sense of optimism must be low, or of computational assumptions that if one scores low on many scores then one's overall score should be low.

Commonly identified dimensions included in the sorts of quality of life scales that emerge from this functionalist approach are:

- Physical concerns (symptoms including pain)
- Functional ability (activity)
- Well-being (may include emotional well-being and that of their family)
- Spirituality
- Social functioning
- Satisfaction with treatment
- Future orientation (plans: sense of hope) (Clinch *et al.* 1998: 84).

The second main approach, the phenomenological/hermeneutic, allows more emphasis on an individual identifying their own values and experiences. This can be achieved via qualitative research including semi-structured interviews, diaries or critical incident analysis. Other approaches have included considering how established psychological research tools, the Repertory Grid technique for example (Thunedborg *et al.* 1993), can help identify areas unique to an individual in such a way as to then facilitate scrutiny of change over time.

Given the system world concerns for measures of health outcomes that can be compared across people with similar illnesses, there has been support for the development of approaches that seek to combine individual domains with scales that can then be scored. There are examples in which open-ended questions are added after a series of scale-based items, for example, questions about what one would choose to do if you had less or no pain (see Tugwell *et al.* 1987). Then there are approaches that seek self-nomination of important areas. A notable example is the Schedule for the Evaluation of Individual Quality of Life (SEIQoL) (O'Boyle *et al.* 1992, 1993). Here, the person identifies the significant areas that contribute to their own quality of life and makes a judgement as to the relative importance of those areas. Changes in the composition, and relative significance, of domains can be examined over time.

There are many other examples of specific quality of life measures drawing on these two overall approaches, as shown in Box 5.5.

Box 5.5 Examples of quality of life measures used in palliative care

Missoula-VITAS Quality of Life Index (MVQOLI). This is focused on people with advanced incurable disease, it is not disease-specific. It is based on five dimensions; symptom, function, interpersonal, well-being, transcendent – plus an overall global quality of life item. It is useful as an assessment tool for patient and health professionals to identify dimensions that need particular intervention (Byock and, Merriman 1998).

McGill Quality of Life Questionnaire (MQOL). A quality of life measure for all patients with life-threatening illness, from diagnosis to cure or death. It assesses general domains including the existential. It balances physical and non-physical concerns and includes positive and negative aspects of quality of life (Cohen *et al.* 1995).

For a review of instruments see Brown University (2005)

These instruments focus on domains of one's life and consider how they interrelate and contribute to an overall sense of quality of life. But one can also approach quality of life from a temporal perspective. Do you focus on years of life, or life in the years? Health conditions, treatment regimes, and projected outcomes combine to generate a dialogue (often an internal one) about how far one would trade off more years of life for fewer years of higher quality life (Lawton *et al.* 1999: see Q-TWIST and time trade-off approaches in Box 5.4). This 'time trade-off' idea has been addressed in the idea of Valuation of Life (VOL) (Lawton *et al.* 1999). This is a mediating construct that brings together a more global concept of quality of life with the impact of considerations of health on desired years of life. There are implications in this idea for suggesting that care planning should ensure it seeks to determine and maximize patient/resident preferences and values 'thereby broadening care plans to include individualized social, spiritual, and other activities that enhance quality of life' (Noelker and Harel 2001: 10). This is an approach that sits close to the palliative care ideal. It also has resonance for discussions about autonomy and advance directives/living wills and euthanasia.

Quality of life in dementia care

There are now many works considering the quality of life of people with dementia (see Lawton 1997; Bond 1999; Albert and Logsdon 2000; Jennings 2000;

Post 2000b; Noelker and Harel 2001; Smith *et al.* 2005). These include engagement with the philosophical and conceptual assumptions of quality of life
measures and the specific challenges raised by dementia, in many instances
related to the idea we have kept returning to, that of personhood (Kitwood
and Bredin 1992b). They also include an engagement with what are appropriate measures (Bond 1999) and with many of the issues about approach and
focus discussed above.

Much of the discussion about quality of life in palliative care is directly relevant
to dementia care – the relative benefits of emphasizing the objective and subjective, with the concomitant questions of what to include and how to weigh
items, as well as how to facilitate comparison across time and between individuals. There are some different areas of emphasis, specifically as Hughes asks,
'once a person is incapable, should quality be judged by reference to how
things are now, or by considerations of what the person would have wanted
based on things they said in the past?' (Hughes 2003: 525). This is a subject we
considered in Chapter 4. Hughes responds to his own question by a challenging review of the conceptual issues that an engagement with quality of life for
people with dementia provoke. He concludes that quality of life, as such, is not
measurable because the concept cannot be bounded. A phenomenological
approach, drawing on the idea of personhood, does offer a route forward via
a consideration of aspects of quality of life that together form parts of our
'situated embodied' selves.

There have been disease-specific instruments developed for people with
dementia.

Brod *et al.*'s (1999a, b) Dementia Quality of Life Instrument (D-QoL) has
been widely used. It has 29 items and was tested on 99 participants with mild
to moderate dementia, of whom 96 per cent were able to respond to questions
appropriately. Its focus is on subjective experience and evaluation of life circumstance. There are four context domains: dementia signs and symptoms,
comorbid illness, physical and social environment, individual characteristics.
There are also functioning and behavioural variables. Five quality of life
domains are presented: aesthetics; positive affect; negative affect, self-esteem,
feelings of belonging. Brod *et al.* concluded (1999a) that persons with mild to
moderate dementia can be considered good informants of their own subjective states. This paves the way to consider patient responses rather than proxy
measures, as had previously been the practice, for assessing quality of life for
persons with dementia.

As we have introduced in our review of DCM, above, the specifics of dementia raise the possibility that an assessment of quality of life and of quality of
care can be carried out using the same instrument. Doing so can overcome

some of the difficulties in accessing either objective or subjective data by considering the whole context of a person's life in a care environment. Such an approach has an added attraction. It can be used to develop intervention programmes to improve those areas that are found to be problematic. That is, it can be of significance both at the level of understanding and as a guide for action. Tobin's (1999) analysis of threats to self in long-term care, offers a further example. This identifies as components of quality: psychosocial care; warmth of staff and resident relationships; availability of personally meaningful activities and stimulation; tolerance for resident deviance such as aggression, wandering, incontinence; extent to which residents are treated as individuals. These components relate to different sorts of coping techniques (techniques used by people struggling to maintain their integrity of the self). Some are 'rational', some less so (see Table 5.3). In relation to the less rational areas it is an approach that identifies those things that staff find particularly hard to deal with. The approach assumes that if staff understood these difficult behaviours as being part of the person's attempts to preserve the self this might both serve to enhance the importance of psychosocial care over the narrow preoccupation with 'technical' efficiency and help reduce the damage to morale that exposure to such behaviour generates.

A strategy to support the 'rational' and to recognize and respond to the 'irrational' provides a guide to action for carers, a means of assessing the quality of the environment and a proxy understanding of quality of life if one assumes a positive value for the rational and a negative for the irrational.

Other measures also engage with the social context of the individual's life. The Alzheimer's Disease-Related Quality of Life instrument (ADRQL) measures social interaction, awareness of self, enjoyment of activities, feeling and mood

Table 5.3 Coping mechanisms to help maintain the integrity of the self (Tobin 1999)

Rational	Less rational
Involved in meaningful activities.	Magical mastery – reality is ignored or denied.
Control over daily activities and interactions.	Verbal and physical aggressiveness under stress.
Contracting one's personal space, sense of future time and range of relationships – for ease of management.	Functional paranoia – blaming others to reduce feelings of vulnerability.
Downwards social comparison – that is, seek out others in one's environment who can be considered worse than oneself.	Acceptance of repressed material.

and response to surroundings (Rabins *et al.* 1999). Lawton (1991) argues that to assess quality of life in a residential establishment one needs to focus on relationships and positive and negative affect in addition to objective measures of the environmental features of the facility. Lawton's approach brings together many of the approaches discussed in this chapter. Set up because of a perceived paucity of information into the needs of residents and a recognition of the wide range of facilities they were cared for in, the Collaborative Studies of Long-Term Care (CS-LTC) programme in the USA (Zimmerman *et al.* 2005) draws on major studies of long-term care. If one looks across such major studies, one can identify considerable differences in the components identified in different research tools to identify aggregate quality of life, and one can see different methods of data collection. 'Because of these differences, correlations between measures are moderate at best, suggesting that multiple indicators are needed to adequately reflect the richness of life' (Zimmerman *et al.* 2005: 6). In the UK Smith *et al.* (2005) have both evaluated current methodologies for measuring health-related quality of life for people with dementia and have developed a new instrument, DEMQOL. The new measure is suitable in mild/moderate and severe dementia and is available in self-completion and proxy completion versions. Its aim is to access via a 28 (or 31 for the proxy measure) item scale the subjective perceptions and experience of people with dementia in such a way that a health-related quality of life score can be identified.

Even people with severe health and functional impairment can show high levels of subjective well-being. Levels of morale, life-satisfaction and subjective health can mediate losses associated with dementia and the impact of those losses on psychological functioning (Heidrich and Ryff 1993). The existence of such subjective concerns might explain why health care providers rate ill older people as having a poorer quality of life than the ratings older people give themselves (Birren and Deutchman 1991).

Conclusion

If we listen to the voices of those whose relatives have dementia, some of the concerns about quality of care and quality of life we have examined in this chapter fade into the background as the quotidian reality of end of life care asserts a different focus. Alan Bennett described the nursing home where his mother lived, sharing a room with three other women with dementia:

> The turnover of residents is quite rapid since whoever is quartered in this room is generally in the last stages of dementia. But that is not what they die of. None of these lost women can feed herself and to feed them properly, to spoon in sufficient mince, and mashed carrot topped off with rhubarb and custard to keep them going, demands

the personal attention of a helper, in effect one helper per person. Lacking such one-to-one care, these helpless creatures slowly and quite respectably starve to death. This is not something anybody acknowledges, nor the matron or the relatives (if, as is rare, they visit) and not the doctor who makes out the death certificate. But it is so.

(Bennett 2005: 114–15)

In this chapter, we have reviewed the ways the system world has identified and privileged an idea of quality as a key dimension in service provision and evaluation. We have identified that an input and process model of quality is generally used to evaluate service provision. The quality of services offered, that is, a measure of what is provided (inputs) and how it is provided (process), is assessed either via comparison with predetermined standards via a number of audit tools or by comparison with what has gone on previously in that establishment, or what goes on in comparable other establishments. Such mechanistic assessments of quality need to be supplemented with understandings of quality that come from those who use services. Attention has been directed to seeking the voice of service users in both palliative care and dementia care of late, but more can be done. Further, there are different constituencies involved in defining what a quality service might consist of. A possible scenario in considering different priorities in quality of life might see people receiving care emphasizing the wish for choice and autonomy over the environment they live in and the services they receive, families and informal carers might be concerned more with safety and with symptom control, staff and regulatory agencies might prioritize meeting targets and standards set externally.

In chronic illness and in end of life care outcome is not easily identified. Externally defined measures such as rates of cure, length of time symptom free, and so on, that can be used in other areas of health care, have been supplanted with scales based on subjective assessments by the person themselves of their quality of life and how this changes over time. Sometimes the domains included in these assessments are identified by the person, sometimes they are pre-decided. Alternatively, and of particular significance in dementia care, there may be judgements, systematized via validated research measures, built on staff observation.

In this chapter we have sought to present the interface between system world concerns about how to use quality in shaping and evaluating services and the subjective views of those receiving services. In so doing we are continuing a theme of the book in terms of bringing different insights together, in exploring interfaces between the system and life-world, between the etic and emic.

The interface between system and life-world is mediated by structures of power. We referred to Foucault's insights into the way structures of power shape both what the system world considers it should and can do and shapes the subjectivity of people within that life-world earlier in this chapter. That is, there are limitations on both modernist reason and individual agency. Others have recognized the symbiotic relationship between socially preferred terms of reference, narrative frameworks and the language of personal accounts (see Garfinkel 1967; Sacks 1974).[2]

Still there may be space in prevailing structures of power, in discourses, to counter prevailing power. Gubrium argues that 'the local and particular continually insinuate themselves to construct differences'. The local and particular interacts with the institutional narrative and with the prevailing discourse revealing that 'The local cultures of ... institutions are an important part of the sources used by participants to convey to themselves and to others who they are, what they were, and what they will become in the future' (Gubrium 2000: 185).

We have, in this chapter, built on themes evident in other chapters in this book. But our focus has been to examine one area, quality, and through that to examine system world assumptions and their resulting actions. The system world is mediated by myriad centres of local power, for example those enshrined in the practice of the professionals who have to put system intentions into practice. This system world approach has been contrasted with life-world assumptions that capture the insights arising from people's subjectivity, often expressed via personal narrative.

We have argued that, however well-meaning attempts to improve care and to measure that improvement are, unless we engage with subjectivity we can neither critique the assumptions the system world brings to, and imposes on, concepts of quality, nor act upon the realization, implied in the quote with which we began the chapter, that my quality may not be the same as yours.

---

[2] It is argued that narratives, personal accounts shaped as stories, not only tell of experience but are a form of life in their own right (Wittgenstein 1953), they are the first and foundational elements of what is known about personal experience (Lyotard 1984). We return to considerations of the importance of narrative in Chapters 6 and 7.

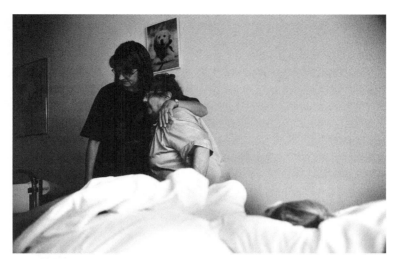
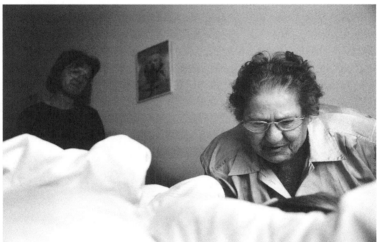
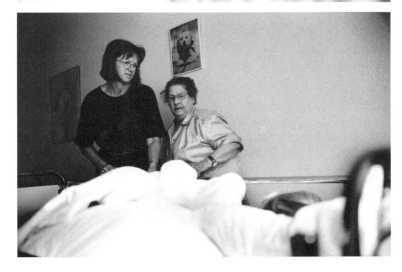

Chapter 6

The good death and dementia

As we grow older
The world becomes stranger, the pattern more complicated
Of dead and living.
T.S. Eliot (East Coker 1944)

Introduction

In a society dominated by doing rather than being, achievement is elevated to
a position where it is axiomatic of what it means to be human: even dying and
death are things we have to be good at. In this chapter we will examine the way
death is defined and we will look at the boundary between living and dying.
We will then go on to examine the idea of the good death. We will argue that in
contemporary Western society what is perceived as a good death takes two
dominant forms – one where death is sudden, but timely, the other where it is
calm, controlled, characterized by making peace with those around you and
being at peace with yourself. The latter is synonymous with the aspirations of
individuals and organizations in the field of palliative care. Neither of these
dominant forms of the good death are readily available to the person with
dementia. It is as if the prevailing mode of what is a good death represents one
final burden for those who have not had the 'good fortune' to die quickly, or to
have had the autonomy, self-control and benefit of skilled and dedicated carers
that would allow them to accord to the peaceful dying ideal.

The good death is a much more complex concept than this contemporary
snapshot reveals. It is not historically fixed – we will briefly summarize how it
has been understood at various points in time. It is contingent upon the point
of view we adopt both as people who die and who care for others who die and
as researchers, practitioners and theorists who engage with 'dying'. It is contingent on the shifting circumstances of our living and of our dying. What is good
about a death will vary according to whose point of view we privilege.

After examining what is a good death we will ask how the palliative care
ideal is compromised by encounters with modernist medicine and utilitarian
social policy. We will suggest that the good death is reframed as a focus on the
'good enough death'. The good death is characteristically engaged with as

a concept located in the individual, but it will look different if we think of a good death interactionally, as a social concept. We will examine what a good death looks like if we consider the focus of concern to be the family, the place a person lives (this might be the neighbourhood of a person's home, or a care home or hospital) or if the focus of concern is on social networks.

Consistent with the approach of the rest of this book we argue that dying and death can be positioned as either a system world or life-world concern. Again, as in previous chapters, we argue that the system world has colonized the life-world in such a way that a good death is best understood as a discourse (a systematized structure of significance supported by, and supporting, social power) rather than a narrative (a subjective account emerging from the lived experience of each individual). To address what might constitute a good death with dementia we will reassert life-world subjectivity, and consider what a system of meaning and care that would emerge if this was done might look like.

Amongst the many views about dying with dementia there is a belief that when death occurs it is a relief to the carers and a release to the person with dementia, whatever the other circumstances of the death. Further, there is a belief that the person had already died, that is, that death was contemporaneous with the onset of dementia, not with physical death. This is sometimes expressed by family and friends describing the person with dementia who has died as being different to the person that they had known and loved. This is a belief that we have examined earlier in relation to understandings of the self (see Chapter 4). These beliefs are located in a system world where dementia is subjected to a widespread therapeutic nihilism (nothing can be done) or marginalization (it is hidden away), and in a life-world where many attitudes to dementia reflect the system world inadequacies in help offered and the prevalence of a discourse that only an autonomous life is a life worth living.

Death is both embodied and social. One dies both physically and socially and in many cases these occur simultaneously. However, many people experience social death a considerable time before physical death. Social death is characteristically a process, it occurs via small steps. Physical death might be assumed to be an event, something occurring once and at a specific time and place, but defining physical death has been controversial and has changed over time. Influencing these changes has been the technology of medical care advances, for example, life-support techniques, and a shifting legislative stance, often tested via litigation. Death is not defined as being the point at which the heart stops beating, or breathing ceases – the life-world or poetic paradigm. It is a debate around death occurring when brain activity ceases that has become central in the system world now – the neurological paradigm. That debate, which assumes brain function to be the thing that defines life, is problematic for advanced dementia. For example, if a person is in a persistent vegetative state they have no brain function, save brainstem activity. This means they have no cognitive, emotional or relation potential. Legally, the confirmation of such a state has permitted the withdrawal of life support systems and hence the end of all brain or body activity. This justifies, in law, defining death based on loss of higher brain activity – but what does loss of higher brain activity mean in the context of considering dementia? In Alzheimer's disease,

> Some neurological events are occurring in the higher brain, no matter how fragmented and limited. Thus, it is impossible to place most, if not all, persons with AD in some other metaphysical category (e.g., 'no longer human').
>
> (Post 2000b: 30)

Post's 'most, if not all' allows him to recognize that some people live long enough with AD to become neurologically vegetative. Does this mean that in such a position life support can be withdrawn because life has ended?

Death as the point at which brain activity ceases is not the accepted definition for all people. The moment of biological death is defined by Sudnow (1967) to be the cessation of cellular activity. However, he suggests that 'clinical death' may also be identified as the appearance of death signs upon physical examination. Here, we have two further possibilities – brain activity measures are too limited, cellular activity assumes functions beyond the brain. But death may also be something that arises from an interaction between a professional and a dying/dead person. That is, the naming of death is what defines death. Perhaps death only occurs when someone in authority says it has occurred. In practice this is the way many of us will experience the moment of death of someone close to us – we will ask, or we will be told, by a professional (doctor or nurse usually) that the person has died.

There are also debates about life ending not based on brain or cellular activity but on a balance between suffering and quality of life. That is, to be alive does not mean one is living – living is a state that is predicated upon a certain level of quality of life. In this debate it is argued that life is considered to have ended if it does not meet a composite but essentially subjective measure. Life, here, is defined as something that encompasses, but goes beyond, the physical/neurological/cellular assumptions about what life is.[1] In the main this

---

[1] The *Oxford English Dictionary* defines life in a number of ways – one definition is that life is the assemblage of the functional activities by which a living animal or plant, or a living portion of organic tissue, can be separated from dead, or non-living matter. It is also defined as a word used to designate a condition of power, activity, or happiness, in contrast to metaphorical 'death'. Life is a word whose etymology allows for these different uses and it would seem important in discussing life, the good life, and ending life to be clear about how far we are emphasizing a functional or metaphorical understanding.

debate is framed in the context of discussions of the centrality of autonomy/ self-determination.

As well as the argument that living is more than being alive, there is also an argument that engages with the more reciprocal concept of a right to life. Here, captured by philosopher Anthony Grayling, this argument claims that a right to life is a right to life of a certain minimum quality, 'mere existence is not an automatic good'. Grayling would also have it that choosing when to die is one of life's great questions and should be left to individual choice – like whom to love and whether to have a family. Problems occur when people have lost their power to express their choice, and did not voice it beforehand: when they were not, as Montaigne would have it, 'booted and spurred, and ready to go'. According to Grayling exercising the right to die requires, 'sound mind and settled purpose'(Grayling 2005; see also Grayling quoted in Smith 2005).

In the UK, there has been much discussion prompted by a parliamentary bill proposed by Lord Joffe (debated in the House of Lords May 2006) which, had it passed, would have permitted assisted dying for the terminally ill. Doctors would have been allowed to provide a patient with the means to commit suicide if a patient asked repeatedly, was competent to make their own decisions and was suffering acutely in the terminal phase of their illness. Baroness Warnock, writing in support of the Joffe bill, said;

> Some would prefer death to the drawn out process of being kept alive and conscious.. especially for those more inclined to think of life as lived by a particular person, the person valued rather than the life itself, it is possible to question whether the sanctity of life is a principle from which parliament can properly derive its decisions.

> (Warnock 2006: 31)

Lord Joffe's Bill did not proceed, but there have been similar initiatives elsewhere in the world (see 1994 Death with Dignity Act, Oregon, USA[2]).

---

[2] The US state of Oregon passed its Death with Dignity Act in 1994. It legalized physician-assisted dying with certain restrictions. It is available to capable adults diagnosed with a terminal illness. The patient has to be confirmed as not suffering from a mental condition impairing judgement. Requests to be prescribed lethal medication have to be made in writing to a physician, confirmed by two witnesses, the terminal illness diagnosis has to be confirmed by a second physician. After a 15-day wait a second oral request has to be made before the prescription is written. By the end of 2005, 246 people had taken their lives under the procedures of the Act. See www.deathwithdignity.org, for the text of the law see www.dhs.state.or.us/publichealth/chs/pas/ors.cfm (both sites accessed 6 February 2007).

These approaches to life and death, clustered as they are around the idea of individual choice, are problematic for those people who are the focus of this book:

- We have discussed how challenging it is to consider accessing the subjectivity of the person with dementia;

- Any judgements based on balancing suffering and quality of life are problematic, both in terms of assessing levels of suffering and measuring quality of life in the group we focus on;

- Setting up a choice system about ending one's life, based on assumptions about sound mind and settled purpose, might meet some people's life-world concerns but it is also a system world issue when it is proposed as integral to a legislative framework defining the parameters of the legally possible. What happens to those who do not meet the criteria for being allowed choice? Surely there is a chance they get consigned to a suboptimum 'sink' facility, as has been the case for those considered beyond effective interventions but in need of continuing care – those with chronic mental illness, frail older people, those with learning disabilities. That is, in a system world, legislative change cannot just be assessed for the potential benefits to those who might avail themselves of the new possibilities. It has also to be assessed in terms of its impact on other parts of the system.

This last point underlines a shortcoming of utilitarian social policy – consider how different it would be if one started from, for example, a position advocated by philosopher John Rawls. His approach begins from a justice perspective (Rawls 1972) and seeks to develop a theory of justice that includes both positive and negative rights (things we need to have for justice to be possible and things we need to be protected from). Any justice system needs to be practical enough to be consistent with the pursuit of individual interests but also convincing enough to those people who may have to make sacrifices to bring the system about. Here, resource allocation would be determined according to the needs of the more vulnerable and not according to the interests of the majority (see Doyal and Gough 1991).

We now turn to two socially constructed discourses which offer insight into understanding the management of death, from both the individual's perspective and a wider societal view. These relate to the nature of the life–death boundary, and the idea of there being a 'good' death.

The boundary between life and death

Life and death are separated in a number of ways in contemporary society (Hockey 1990). Markers of separation may be categorized spatially, socially and temporally. The spatial separation of life and death occurs when institutions become key places for death to take place in. Even if not dying within the walls of an institution, the institution may enter a person's home, through, for example, health and social care staff visiting the home of a dying person. Social boundaries exist, through the marginalization of older, dying and bereaved people. There is also a temporal boundary which determines the right time to die – when one is old. However, the life–death boundary may appear to be less clearly defined if one looks from the perspective of the dying person.

Improved social conditions, alongside medical advances in public health and curative medicine, have eradicated many of the killers of the last century. For example, the availability of antibiotics has reduced rates of death from the 'old man's friend' pneumonia. Consequently, more people live longer, and develop chronic conditions which have to be managed for increasingly extended periods of time. Although biological death may have been delayed in many areas, social death appears to be encroaching on more people. Mulkay and Ernst (1991) expressed the view that, with the current rational organization of death, the relationship between social and biological death has been redrawn in unexpected ways. Increased medical knowledge and more sophisticated diagnostic tests ensure that in many cases it is possible to foresee death at an early stage of the illness. An individual's death may also be postponed via technological intervention, although they may be subject to marginalization and social death for lengthy periods as a consequence (Moller 1990). The area of technological innovation and its impact on death promises to raise many conceptual, practical and emotional challenges in the future. For example, the identification of particular genes linked with serious or life-limiting conditions, like Huntington's chorea, raises the possibility of a lifetime living with a sense of the possibilities of premature death. Secondly, the possibilities of organ replacement, not just by other people's organs but by mechanical devices, offers the possibility of the emergence of cyborg bodies and, with this, the need to rethink what a living body is. There is even an engagement with the possibility that science can make the ancient dream of the possibilities of immortality come to pass (Appleyard 2007).[3]

---

[3] Appleyard reports on scientists who are allied with the 'life-extension movement' and the proponents of 'medically immortality'. Their thesis is that there is no reason why our bodies should be allowed to fall apart and stop working: nano technology for example might allow our bodies to cleared out of accumulated rubbish and repaired where required. He locates such discussions in a history of ideas of immortality and he considers how far immortality might both be personally undesirable and might kill culture. He considers that culture has taken the shape it has because it has been fashioned as a response to death. He does summarize how one might prolong life by quoting an unnamed teacher who advises students, 'Be nice, be thin and have daughters' (Appleyard 2007: 235).

The implications of a social death have also been considered by Sudnow (1967) and Glaser and Strauss (1965, 1968), drawing on Goffman's concept of the non-person, and the consequences of social withdrawal for the individuals so defined. Goffman defines non-persons as 'standard categories of persons who are sometimes treated in their presence as if they were not there' (Goffman 1959: 152). Although bodily present, these people are marginalized and rendered invisible. Within a hospital setting, Glaser and Strauss identified social death as something that follows the recognition that a patient is dying clinically: the patient's involvement in social life is restricted by their geographical isolation in the hospital, and by their voluntary or involuntary withdrawal from social relationships. A similar process accompanies the movement of an older person into a residential or nursing home (Hockey 1990; Mulkay and Ernst 1991; Froggatt 2001), or a person being referred to a hospice (see Lawton 2000). In effect it is the public perception of these establishments as places people go to die, however partial a description this may be, that triggers the assumption that there physical death is near and that enhances their social death.

Mulkay and Ernst (1991) and Mulkay (1993) give another definition of social death: the cessation of the individual as an active agent in other people's lives. It is possible that an individual may be physically dead, but still influence the actions of the survivors, either through legal documents such as wills, or through their lingering, influential personalities. For example in popular entertainment, films such as the Hollywood production *Ghost* and the British film produced in the 1990s, *Truly, Madly, Deeply* focused on a relationship which continued after one partner had died. The success of such films perhaps reveals the wide currency of this notion, one found in tales of ghosts and the supernatural across centuries. We might see the ghost of the murdered King in Shakespeare's *Hamlet* as an earlier example. Such examples show that an interactional process may be evident beyond physical death (Bloch and Parry 1982).[4] It is surely commonplace that one takes cognisance of the continued

....

4 There are mythical stories about returns from the land of the dead. The story of Orpheus and Eurydice has Orpheus travelling to the Underworld to bring back his dead wife, Eurydice – the one condition the Gods made was that he must not look back as he brought her out. He did – anxious to be sure she was following him – and as he had broken his agreement with the Gods, Eurydice had to remain in the land of the dead (see Grant 1998: 200). There are, of course, stories of resurrection central to the Christian tradition. In non-Christian contemporary literature, Philip Pullman in *The Amber Spyglass* (Pullman 2001), Volume 3 of *His Dark Materials*, explores ideas of 'rescue' from the land of the dead. The idea of a miraculous rescue, either via the intermediary of faith or science, is an often present but frequently hidden feature of many people's encounters with 'incurable' illness.

presence of the dead in the life of the living; what would they have thought of this, would they have approved of that, and so on.

In a newspaper interview the writer Martin Amis discussed the illness and death of his friend, novelist Saul Bellow: 'He had Alzheimer's and sometimes it was painful. But when someone dies, you're not in a situation, you're in a process' (Cooke 2006). Humphreys (1981) defines this process of dying as encompassing the time from the realization, usually by others, that someone is dying, to the complete cessation of all social actions directed towards their remains, including their entombment (burial or cremation). She argues for the extension of our understanding of the period of death in this way because of the many different types of losses associated with a person's death. For example, there is the loss of an individual, upon the physical death of the person, but also the perceived loss of identity or personhood, which occurs with social death. Three groups of people have been identified as having the likely attribution of being seen as socially dead (Sweeting and Gilhooly 1991–1992, 1997): very old people, those individuals at the end stage of a long-term chronic illness, and people who are perceived to have lost their personhood, akin to Goffman's notion of the non-person (Goffman 1959). Older people with dementia fall into all of these categories, thus compounding the likelihood of their being seen as socially dead.

It can also be observed that people other than the dying, through their association with death, can be socially marginalized. This might include the bereaved or even those people caring for the dying.

For the dying and their family carers, the boundary between life and death is fluid. It is a zone of transition, or oscillation. There is a moving back and forward around death, whether death is seen functionally or metaphorically. Armstrong adds the point that:

> It is necessary to be nominalist about death. Death is not a thing or event existing independently of human consciousness; it is simply the word given to a certain threshold, interface, space or point of separation.

(Armstrong 1987: 655)

When social death is a characteristic shared by a category of people (here people with dementia) we see two accompanying practices. The first is sequestration – these people are hidden away and strong barriers are created between them and their former world. The second is that they are subjected to close monitoring and control within the sequestrated space. These are twin characteristics typical of prisons and asylums, they are also present in the care of the dying. Disintegrating dying bodies are hidden away in hospices (Lawton 2000), ageing incontinent bodies are managed in care homes (Froggatt 2001) and disintegrating minds are set apart in both and in psychiatric hospitals (Oliver 1999).

Box 6.1 Structural control in residential settings

- Temporal
- Physical
- Material
- Organizational
- Behavioural and linguistic

(Oliver 1999)

Oliver (1999) identifies five areas of structural control present in residential settings that are used to conceal, contain and control the potential disorder arising from the presence of dementia (Box 6.1) Although based on work in one UK residential setting, there are similar accounts to be found in studies of US nursing homes (Pateniti 2003; Gass 2004; Lidz *et al.* 1992).

Reflecting the ways in which the life–death boundary is managed, as described earlier in the chapter, we see here the different ways in which disorder of another type is managed. Temporal control of people with dementia living in a residential setting occurs through the ways in which daily activities are arranged into a routine that ensures a consistency to activity through set mealtimes, drug rounds and other social activities. This regime is operationalized at a collective rather than an individual level. The individual is expected to fit in.

The way physical control occurs in residential settings can be illustrated by the arrangements governing who is allowed in and out. The use of locked doors at the entrance ensures visitors are screened and residents cannot exit without being accompanied. Within settings there are areas with differential access to different groups of residents. Material concealment of the institutional limitations on individuals occurs through the use of 'homely' decor and names for units within the setting, The tensions between being a home for people as well as a place where intimate nursing care is given is an ongoing one that nursing homes have to manage (Froggatt 2001). Organizational control occurs through processes of reporting that downplays unusual events such as illness or death. The decisions about how time is used and structured and the volume of work undertaken by individual care staff (Gass 2004) also serves to make intimate relationships more difficult to develop. The way in which residents are categorized, a practice observed over many years in the care for older people (Evers and Meier 2002) serves to make individuals manageable. Infantilization in the use of language also occurs and it is evident that this is utilized to manage the deterioration observed (Hockey 1990; Hockey and James 1993).

The presence of social death ascribed to people with dementia and their physical segregation shapes the nature of the transition from life to death that they make, which in turn influences the way in which their death is perceived.

A good death

As we said in our opening comments in this chapter, there is not one prevailing societal construct of a good death. Rather, there is a bifurcation between an adherence to the idea that a good death is a sudden death, occurring in an otherwise fit old age and a recognition that, if one is ill, then the aspiration should be that one 'does not suffer'. The sudden death 'ideal' is captured in Roger McGough's 1967 poem (McGough 1983), 'Let me die a young man's death' which includes the iconic lines summarising his wish to be, 'mown down at dawn by a bright red sports car on my way home from an allnight party'. Alternatively, the sudden death ideal is captured in the idea of an active older person moving from a full engagement in the world to a peaceful death – with no intervening incapacity. Richard Hoggart's rueful musings before his shaving mirror capture the element of fantasy/wish fulfilment in this:

> During your morning ablutions, you think of several things you need to do today and by the time you're finished at the wash basin they are gone. You console yourself that Titian was painting at 88, Adenauer running Germany at 87, Alistair Cooke broadcasting weekly at 95, John Gielgud still acting a month before he died at 96 ... James Agate tells the story of Clemenceau on his 80th birthday catching sight of a pretty girl and exclaiming, 'Oh to be 70 again!'
>
> (Hoggart 2006)

If one is not to die suddenly and without illness, then a further construct of the good death is captured in what has been termed the 'revivalist' discourse of palliative care (see Seale 1998; Clark 2002). This combines the achievement of practical objectives: optimum symptom control, social network assumptions: the close involvement of family/friends, and assumptions about individual agency: the dying person at the centre of a care network whose priorities they set themselves.

The possibility of questioning a generally identified preference to die quickly is made possible by better symptom control and resonates with a wish to exercise control over (even) the end of life. One cancer expert (a doctor) talks about a slow death in Kfir and Slevin (1991: 53):

> I can actually see a lot of advantages, an advantage in having a chance to be able to come to terms with dying and with yourself, other people, to sort things out in your life over a period of time: to round off your life.

In the interviews Young and Cullen undertook in London's East End with people near the end of their life, and with their carers, other constructs, also with some social resonance, are revealed. These include different strategies adopted by the dying; the fighters, 'who held on with such admirable tenacity to the small pleasures of life, and the consolations of their own spirits'; the accepters (the older ones in the study) who absorbed themselves in memories of the past, reviewing their earlier life. Some sought to put right what they saw as the errors of the past (Young and Cullen 1996: 181). What Young and Cullen are presenting also has abiding meaning for the idea of a good death. This seems to include the idea of 'dying work' – of tasks the dying need to address in order to achieve a good death.

Ideas like Hoggart's about the characteristics of a desirable old age and the sudden death, revivalist and dying work constructs are challenged by the intrusions of any mental incapacity and are not able to accommodate the experience of the dementias. As we said in the introduction to this chapter, what is widely assumed to constitute a 'good death' varies over time and across cultures. It also varies according to the age of the person dying and the circumstances of their lives, including the nature of their illness. It may be that the way a good death is perceived by the person who is dying depends on the stage of progression they have reached and the quotidian experiences of living with the demands of an illness: if my pain is particularly bad on one day I may construct my 'good death' differently than I had the day before.

Death has an individual, a local, a social and a symbolic dimension and deciding what is a good death will vary according to which dimension we are considering. Which dimension takes precedence offers insight into the social position of the person who is dying and the prevalent approach to death in society. A good death is also subject to variations in system world power differentials, for example different professions may have incorporated into their culture of practice varied assumptions, both tacit and overt, about what is a good death. The actions they engage in and the options they consider will be shaped by their culture of practice.

The very idea of there being a good death and the possibility of its incorporation into a wider social or professional ideology may lead to the identification of good and bad patients, judged by how far they act in accord with a good death ideal, and it may prompt attempts by caregivers to shape experiences to conform to the good death process. Hart *et al.* (1998) argue that the ideology of the good death legitimates a new form of social control – there is a socially approved dying and death proscribed by normalized behaviours and choices. The ideology dominates the social management of dying and death within the hospice movement (and increasingly so within the broader community), and powerfully constrains the choices of dying people.

Hart *et al.* argue that this ideology of the good death has evolved from the work of French historian Aries, via the work describing clinical practice shaped into the stage theory of reactions to the experience of one's dying of Kübler-Ross (1969). While, in principle, it includes the possibility of a variety of ways of experiencing death, there remains a core element of the ideology comprising dying with dignity, peacefulness, preparedness, awareness, adjustment and acceptance (Hart *et al.* 1998).

Hence an appropriate question in considering a good death is to ask, 'Good death for whom?' Of specific relevance for dementia is a consideration of the centrality given to the views of the person with dementia. That is, is there a point where the views of others, family carers, for example, rise to prominence in dementia and does this differ from the experience in other end of life scenarios?

The palliative care ideology of the good death, as described by Hart, has the potential to replace, in the West at least, *Ars Moriendi,* the art of dying. The art of dying evolved at a time when the only reasonable attitude to the approach of death was to let it happen. While one could do nothing about the symptoms that would lead to one's death, with their appearance it was possible to seek to die in the best way possible. For many this meant to die at peace with God. Now in the developed world, for many, death comes later and more slowly.

> The greatest triumph of the century is to have added twenty-five years to the average expectation of life or, to put it another way, subtracted twenty-five years from the expectation of death.

> (Young and Cullen 1996: 1)

But this 'triumph' carries with it the arrival of 'slow death' – both large numbers of people who, because of their age and frailty, live with the contemplation of their own deaths and more people dying slowly from specific diseases. As Young and Cullen so vividly put it, 'More of the living are dying' (Young and Cullen 1996: 175).

Different ways of thinking about what is a good death can be identified if we look at the historical evolution of the concept. Other differences are better examined via considering contemporary assumptions. We will briefly review arguments that identify changing conceptions of the good death in three periods of history – pre-modern/modern/postmodern. We will then comment in more detail on two areas. First, we will critically review the stance of modern medicine in relation to death and the good death and, secondly, we will examine in some detail the good death in palliative care. We will then go on to argue that we can see a good death as located in social networks – an approach that moves us forward from a more prevalent individualistic focus. That idea of social networks capturing what constitutes a good death will then lead us to consider if there is a viable societal construct of a good death.

Changing perceptions of death in society

Historical differences

There are a number of ways in which changing views of dying and death have been examined. These characteristically take the form of dividing history into phases in which certain ideas have been prevalent and then charting the changes in these dominant ideas, and the consequent influence they exert on understandings of dying and death. Crucial to these models has been the identification of the impact of modernism and, in particular, the rise of reason and science. Reason and science are seen as quintessential to the conceptualization of scientific medicine which, in turn, is portrayed as the epitome of modernism.

It is not our intention to summarize the excellent histories that have engaged with the changing perceptions of death in society.[5] Rather, we will pick out some key issues and debates that are particularly pertinent for our exploring the good death in dementia.

Hiding death away

In the modern era, death, in Ariès term, is tamed (Ariès 1974). It is desacralized, transformed into a secular event, amenable to human manipulation (Madan 1992). It is repressed in terms of social awareness, that is, death is hidden. Walters summarizes that a good death does not happen yet, is not seen to happen and happens without my noticing it (Walters 2004: 405).

Much of the pre-modern and early modern discussion of death engaged with the significance of death for the life lived, and for the life to come. Death provided a focus for reflection on the meaning of life both for individuals and for society. In effect, death confirmed the order of the world. But the assumptions of modernity include a belief that people should strive for mastery over the world. In this context each death has the capacity to dislodge, to a greater or lesser extent, the ability to believe in the possibility of this mastery. Hence in pre-modern society death confirms order and in modernity death subverts the order of the world (see Seale 1998). The consequence is that in modernity we seek to tame or hide away death. In so doing, we also lose the capacity of death to prompt question about life's meaning. A medicalized dying, shunted to the realm of experts and bounded by technology, does not

---

[5] Philippe Ariès published three books exploring different dimensions of this subject (Ariès 1974, 1981, 1985). His view of death in modern times was influenced by Gorer (1965). There have been publications which take a disciplinary focus – Fulton and Bendiksen (1994), Kastenbaum (1995), Walter (1993). Other key writers are cited in the text.

promote existential questions but is more likely to lead to technical challenges such as those that prompt us to ask, 'could more have been done?' With this substitution of a technical challenge for an existential question death is seen as evidence of a failure and not the culmination of a life.

There are two, apparently different, ways society can ignore the challenge of death. First, by hiding death away and, secondly, by trying everything one can to prevent death happening. The dying can be consigned to a liminal world of the 'not yet dead' (see Glaser and Strauss 1965, 1968). They are set apart, sequestrated. Or they can become the object of 'heroic' intervention, subjected to the belief that every cause of death is something to be resisted, postponed, avoided (see Bauman 1992). To die is a failure of some system, or is a sign of a moral flaw in the person dying. This approach can promote a tendency towards futile treatment – futile meaning with low probability of having any effect, or producing an effect that is of no benefit to the patient (see Seymour 2001 on the challenge to be faced if medical technology is to coexist with dignified dying).

We suggested that these two approaches were only apparently different ways to respond to death. What unites them is an implicit stance towards the person who is dying that objectifies and depersonalizes them. We have examined in previous chapters both the sequestration of people with dementia and the likelihood of their being subjected to futile treatment (or to too little treatment – effectively displaying the same lack of person-centredness.) With dementia there is a compounding and perverse assumption that social death (due to an assumed lack of intellectual capacity) precedes actual death, sometimes by many years, and that the 'actual death' may be constructed in professional and popular discourse as 'a welcome release' – an end to having to live with the 'irrational'. That is, we can argue that the challenge to the modern is the dementia and not the death – because the person with dementia has become the already dead.[6] Linda Grant in her book about her mother's dementia called this 'the crepuscular realm between life and death' (Grant 1998: 213). It is not just the likely incidence and prevalence of dementia in an ageing society that explains the arrival of dementia as *the* dread disease for the twenty-first century in the West, it is it the absence of reason, coupled with the absence of an effective 'technical' response to it.

---

[6] Foucault (1967) argues that the mentally ill person had replaced the leper as the already dead of society. The strongest contemporary candidates to take over this role were people with AIDS but, with the advent of new treatments for them, the strongest candidates are now people with dementia.

The contemporary significance of the points made about the challenge death poses to modernity and its assumptions of control, and about the particular way that dementia may pose a similar challenge, are called into question if we accept that we have moved into a world best characterized as postmodern. This allows us to consider that one can have a model of a good death built around the flexibility of choosing one's own way of dying (Walter 1994). The paradox in postmodern assumptions is to believe that in a world where all choices are possible that all people can choose.[7] Any model of a good death held by an influential group will exert a power on the person having to make choices (Hart *et al.* 1998).

Geographic mobility and cultural heterogeneity mean that we often encounter 'cultural and moral strangers'. When we do this, the dangers of imposing one's assumption on others is great (Toscani *et al.* 2003: 13). One can be a cultural and moral stranger because one comes from a society that is not well understood by those around you, the Muslim person in a predominantly Christian care home, for example, or you can become a cultural and moral stranger because those caring for you do not try, or are not able, to glimpse your subjective world.

Both social systems and subjectivities are shaped by the prevailing discourse

We cannot assume that anyone involved in providing care to people at the end of their lives is acting other than in ways directed by surrounding ideas, and we can assume that one set of ideas – believed to be evidence-based and to represent an objective truth – will one day be overturned by a shift in the shape of the prevailing discourse (see Box 6.2). When this happens, what we now see as the epitome of reason becomes the outmoded mistakes of the past. [8]

....

[7] The person with dementia is most often constrained in all the choices they make. Their space is bounded, sometimes they are also physically constrained, even bound. Paradoxically, they might in their lack of a past, lack of fixed point of reference and rapidly changing focus exhibit some quintessential signs of being a postmodern person. Being a person without ties may be terrifying as well as exciting. In the past, and in other cultures, people who we now describe as having dementia may have been seen as visionary, as possessed of a spirit perceived to have a deeper wisdom about the nature of life.

[8] Foucault argued that what we understand as rational, as objective and as scientific, is not fixed. It changes over time. New domains of rationality are constituted and old assumptions discarded. Foucault seeks to undermine the importance of both reason and agency, for him these are 'two sides of the same system of thought' (Foucault 1972: 12). That is, neither social practice or individual choice exist outside of the power structures of the prevailing discourse.

Box 6.2 Example of a shift in prevailing ideas: the importance of controlling pain

While there has been a long history of the 'heroic ideal of an individualistic, self-controlled death', evident for example in ancient Greece and Rome (Seale and van der Geest 2004) there has also been a phase in history – now categorized as the pre-modern – in which to die well was seen as to die at peace with one's God and with one's neighbours. Being free from physical pain, in this formulation, requires complex consideration. It is not, in itself, an assumed good. Indeed, evidence of suffering might enhance the value of one's death in the sight of God and of one's neighbours. One might aspire to die in 'Raptures of holy joy' (Walters 2004: 405). The original aim of hospices was to bring the dying person to the right relationship with God: medical skills were secondary.

Medicine and the good death

We have argued above that medicine is intrinsically linked to the modern and its science and that dying is seen as a challenge within this paradigm (Kleinman 1995). This is eloquently described by Nuland, drawing on his own clinical experiences as a surgeon in the United States:

> We live today in the era not of the art of dying, but of the art of saving life, and the dilemmas in that art are multitudinous. As recently as half a century ago, that other great art, the art of medicine, still prided itself on its ability to manage the process of death, making it as tranquil as professional kindness could. Except in the too-few programs such as hospice, that part of the art is now mostly lost, replaced by the brilliance of rescue and, unfortunately, the all too common abandonment when rescue proves impossible ... (for some enthusiastic doctors) death is an implacable enemy. To such warriors, even a temporary victory justifies the laying waste of the fields in which a dying man has cultivated his life.
>
> (Nuland 1997: 265)

Nuland continues by pointing out that many of the resulting victories are pyrrhic, not worth the suffering they brought with them, and that they are often pursued because of the drive of the doctor and not the wishes of the patient and the family whose support and consent may appropriately be seen as clutching at straws of possibility held out for them.

Nuland's points are reminiscent of Illich's (1976) critique of the medicalization of dying. Illich argued that it produced:

- A loss of the capacity to accept death and suffering as meaningful aspects of life,
- A state of total war against death at all stages of the life cycle,
- A crippling of personal and family care and devaluing of the traditional rituals surrounding dying and death.

Illich sought to demonstrate

the paradoxically counterproductive effectiveness implicit in disproportionate techniques … clinical, social, and cultural iatrogenesis; namely the production of multifaceted misery. [For him the medical establishment is] an enterprise claiming, in effect, to abolish the need for the art of suffering by a technically engineered pursuit of happiness … the pursuit of happiness is translated into the pursuit of 'health'.

(Illich 1995: 8)

Ros Levenson's (2004) account of her mother's dementia and her hospitalization provides a vivid confirmation of Illich's position. Her mother was 83, had dementia and her final hospital stay lasted 28 days.

The worst aspects of this sad chapter were a result of professional defensiveness, which at times overrode my mother's needs, her known wishes, and a presumed ethos of multidisciplinary working to meet her needs. It was truly horrible to have to deal with a nurse who lamented that she would have to fill in incident forms if things went wrong. I felt sorry that she felt so unsupported that she had to make this my problem, but it was inappropriate and unacceptable behaviour, and it came my way when I felt least like dealing with it.

Levenson (2004: 1244)

Many of the problems related to how far her mother could be fed by mouth and the proposed insertion of a PEG (percutaneous gastrostomy tube):

Many of the nurses and some of the doctors found it hard to stop short of maximum intervention to prolong life. But in the openness of a public ward where patients and visitors see and share so much of what is going on, the ordinary people in and around the beds seemed to see it differently. Professionals in health care need to remember that there is more to life than being kept alive, and dying need not become a medical event.

(Levenson 2004: 1244)

Palliative care and the good death

Nuland (1997) identified that hospice programmes were one place where the art of medicine was still practiced, and we have summarized the revivalist discourse identifying the good death in palliative care. However, the palliative care approach exists within the broader context of societal expectations and professional assumptions. It is not immune to the same pressures that produce the modernist medical approach we have identified as being so flawed in relation to end of life care. In this section we will examine some of the tensions within which palliative care exists.

Sandman (2005) identifies several features of the good death in palliative care which exemplify attributes that come together to create a good death. A good death comprises:

- Facing death. This encompasses acquaintance, awareness and acceptance of death. This leads, Sandman argues, to self-possession in the face of suffering.

- Preparations for death. This includes a consideration of the rituals one wishes to have, a completion of worldly affairs, an end of life review and the possible of planning the detail of one's dying.

- Considering different aspects of the environment that surround the death include the extent to which it is peaceful, how far it is public and how the presence of technology is handled.

It is as if palliative care staff see death as good when the components of the palliative care approach have been achieved – symptom control achieved, care taken over the relational and social context, an appropriate setting and appropriate persons present, completed preparation by the dying person and a sense of existential well-being arrived at (see Sandman 2005; Singer *et al.* 1999; Turner *et al.* 1996; Payne *et al.* 1996; Toscani *et al.* 2003).

Tensions are possible between the views of patients, relatives and staff inculcated in the palliative care approach. That tension emerges from a possible different construction put upon the good death from these different parties – for example, the patient may prioritize awareness, the relatives pain control and the staff the achievement of the components of the revivalist good death in palliative care. There are also likely to be pressures to both move the palliative care approach nearer to the modernist orthodoxy and to codify its practices such that it becomes a discourse defining how a person should die, rather than a template revealing the scope of the possible.

If it is not death that is seen as failure but rather the failure is dying without the control of symptoms, and if these symptoms are defined broadly (with mental and spiritual anguish deemed appropriate domains for palliation), then there is a danger that bringing these domains into the sphere of legitimate concern for health professionals will lead to the imposition of a rigid regime that implements this good dying. That is, there will be a protocol about what one should do and institutional cultures, professional assumptions and a strong sense of peer pressure will try to choreograph a model of good dying. Perhaps something that is polite, conformist, reconciled – a sort of constructed serenity 'lace curtain dying'. Dylan Thomas's entreaty, 'Do not go gentle into that goodnight / Old age should burn and rave at close of day'[9] if acted upon would be considered deviant behaviour or responded to as pathology.

Examples of the areas where a palliative care orthodoxy might impact include:

- Suffering comes to be seen as a problem to be solved – to be dealt with via the interventions of the symptomatologists of 'just another specialty' of palliative care (Clark 2002; see Kearney 1992).
- A form of social control develops in which the rejection of 'patienthood' by dying or bereaved people is labelled as a form of deviance' (Clark 2002).

In the related context of bereavement care, stage theories, or illustrative models, like for example Kübler-Ross's (1969) stages of loss, can be implemented in a prescriptive way rather than as a descriptive device (see Walter 1999: 161–2[10]).

Clark has summed up the implications of these possibilities for a new orthodoxy by observing that there is a tendency/danger that; 'the putative "holism" of palliative care philosophy masks a new, more subtle form of surveillance of dying and bereaved people in modern society' (Clark 2002; see Clark and Seymour 1999).

Good enough dying

McNamara has argued that there has been a shift in hospice practice and in the prevailing ethos of care from one characterized by a model of a 'good death' to one of a 'good enough death'. Hospices re-introduced a ritual for dying in a context where it was disappearing. This ritual depended on open communication and an acceptance of death by both the person who was dying and by those caring for them. However, she argues, this 'has become increasingly inappropriate in the current climate of patient autonomy and consumer choice' (McNamara 2004: 929). It is also increasingly difficult to sustain in the context of 'an increasing institutionalization of hospice care (which) may compromise

---

[9] Walters refers to Spanish novelist and philosopher Miguel de Unamuno who sees a sense of struggle as the approach that brings fulfilment and meaning. One should live with contradictions rather than assuming one can reconcile the wish to live and the inevitability of death. (see Walters 2004: 407–8). Unamuno says that not wanting to die but knowing we will is a conflict between will and reason that cannot be resolved. It is a paradox because it involves conflicting parts of our humanity. We love life 'with a profound experience of struggle'. 'It is precisely this sense of struggle, which marks us out as human and this, rather than serenity, which brings fulfilment to our life and meaning to our death.' Unamuno asks, 'May God give you glory – but not peace'.

[10] See Simonds and Rothman (1992) for a discussion of the way the bereaved interpret the processes of grief and bereavement.

the movement's founding ideals' (McNamara *et al.* 1994: 1501). That institutionalization is linked to:

1. An encroachment of medicine (Clark 2002),

2. A routinization characteristic of many movements that are initiated by charismatic leaders (James and Field 1992),

3. A medical technological imperative to treat (or to palliate) (McNamara *et al.* 1994),

4. The challenges put upon the movement consequent on its rapid expansion (Abel 1986).

There may also be changes prompted by the characteristics of the patients being referred for hospice care or specialist palliative care. The severity of symptoms may be greater now that generalist palliative care has developed in expertise and in availability. More straightforward matters that once might have been cared for by specialists can be dealt with by the now better-informed generalists. The average length of stay in hospice and specialist palliative care units appears to be reducing. This is due to a combination of pressure of numbers and finance-led anxiety on the part of those organizations charged with funding care – in the UK these are Primary Care Trusts. One implication of more severe symptoms and shorter lengths of stay is that it is more difficult for staff to get to know the whole person. In such a situation they may feel it is a justifiable focus and aspiration to control the patient's pain (Lawton 2000). Clark (2002) cites two revealing studies:

1. A US study describing dying patients as 'caught up in a medical juggernaut driven by a logic of its own, one less focussed on human suffering and dignity than on the struggle to maintain vital functions' (Moskowitz and Nelson 1995: 53–55).

2. An Australian study which identified 24 problem areas in an inpatient palliative care setting that prompted interventions from staff. All but two were physical rather than psychosocial or spiritual in type – the two exceptions were depression and delirium (Good and Stafford 2001).

Returning to McNamara, her conclusion is that a capacity to alleviate symptoms has been prioritized over other aspects of the original hospice alliance of physical, psychosocial and spiritual care, and in so doing the good death has been replaced by the good enough death.

Moving beyond the individual

In Table 6.1, we contrast the end of two iconic lives. Both deaths were the result of sentences imposed by the State. For one, the time was chosen and the

Table 6.1 Two iconic lives

Socrates	Jesus
Good death	Bad death
No anxiety about dying – welcomes the release of the soul from the body.	Unpleasant facts of death
	Not wanting to die at this time and in this way,
With his friends	but agreed to accept that his death was, 'not as I
Although sentenced to death – he	will, but as thou wilt' Matthew 26, 39.
chooses when to take the poison.	Feels abandoned by his friends and by God.
See Plato: *The Death of Socrates*	Cries from the cross 'My God my God, why
	hast thou forsaken me?' Mark 15, 34.
	See Mark's gospel.

Adapted from Walters (2004).

death welcome. The other was more anguished. We see how in the Christian tradition death is not supposed to be easy.

So far, in this chapter, we have examined understandings of the life–death boundary and changing conceptualizations of a good death. We have focused on the point of view of the individual who is dying and his, or her, points of contact with those providing care, particularly the medical profession and palliative care providers. We will now shift focus to, first, the individual in their more immediate social context and then to the potential of considering a societal dimension to the good death. Looking at the social in this way will allow us to turn full circle, given that we began by reviewing the way societal attitudes shape understandings about death and give shape to individual beliefs. In contrasting the deaths of Socrates and Jesus, we note that the support of friends in the former and the sense of abandonment by friends in the latter are integral to the experience.

Young and Cullen, in their 1996 book *A good death: conversations with East Londoners*, move the discussion about what is a good death into a dimension that further underlines the sociality of the dying and of death. They identify five things that contribute to making a death a 'good death':

1. 'The goodness was more obvious for people who died a social death,'[11] especially if relationships were close and harmonious.

---

[11] Here a social death means one carried our in close proximity to family, friends and neighbours. It is the opposite of the way social death was used above where the expression was used to identify imposed isolation.

2. 'The good that people do lasts after them: it certainly lasts, and on the whole to their benefit, through a long illness ... a good death emerges from a good life' (1996: 176).

3. 'There seems to be at work around death a peculiar and harsh principle of justice' (1996: 176). That is, those with close and loving relationships that are sustained have more to lose, as do their survivors. So – a good death involves more heartache for the dying and bereaved. 'Pain is the sacrifice that love imposes, especially on the survivors' (1996: 177).

4. The more that can be done for the carers/survivors the better for the dying – so a good death is one where all are taken care of.

5. Both for the dying and their carers the sense of a presence of a wider community appears to contribute to a good death.

There is also the dimension of spiritual needs and relationships. If the spiritual is a key dimension of the holistic care associated with the good death, then the proper practice of religious observance at the end of life is going to be a necessary component of a good death for many people – for example, confession and the administering of the last rites for Catholics.

A good death for people with dementia

In considering the end of life experience of people with dementia, we may find:

◆ A 'social death' preceding actual death (here social death refers to the negative isolation identified by Glaser and Strauss and others). Even if physical death is sudden, it is likely that the person will have lived with social death for some time.

◆ A misconception that dementia takes away the potential of the person to be creative or to be socially engaged, to be charming or whimsical, through the last phase of their life.

◆ Dying that is often protracted in the sense that there appears a remorseless loss of capacities and accretion of health problems.

◆ Difficulty being sure optimum symptom control has been achieved.

◆ Social networks that often exhibit both a considerable level of exhaustion and a pessimism that any positive therapeutic intervention can be achieved.

◆ An assumption that the person with dementia lacks the capacity to express preferences and to feed back assessments of experience.

Each of these assumptions have been considered in various sections of this book. Here, we consider the wider question as to how one might imagine a good death for people with dementia. If one considers the prevailing paradigms of sudden, or of controlled and easeful death, with full engagement until the very end, then one might conclude that people with dementia are excluded from the category of people for whom that there might be a good death. This counsel of despair can be engaged with in the same way that we have approached living until you die with dementia in other areas of this book – namely:

- The identification of bad practice that makes a difficult situation worse,
- Highlighting good practice,
- Critiquing how we understand the self and how we conceptualize care.

As has been our intention throughout this book, we approach this via the twin devices of considering the subjectivity of the person with dementia and considering how to prioritize the life-world over the system world.

Choosing the manner of your death with dementia

In a study of older people asked about making end of life decisions in advance of dementia, most respondents chose the 'low-tech' options. Three-quarters said they would refuse cardiopulmonary resuscitation, ventilation and any form of medically assisted feeding were they to become even mildly demented. Once severely dementia and unable to recognize loved ones, two-thirds of respondents said they would rather die than be hospitalized and be given antibiotics (Gjerdingen *et al.* 1999: 421–5). However, if such intentions were used to shape advance directives about future care provision, problems are encountered, as we examined in Chapter 4, when we considered the possible shifting nature of the self. Once a person has dementia, they may have, 'embraced his handicapped existence with a will to live' (Hertogh 2004a: 394). There is a paradox in saying the person with dementia has become a different person and also saying that they are bound by what was decided in an advance directive. Hence, the crucial issue in engaging with the idea of choice in dementia is both one of capacity and autonomy and also, when considering advance directives, of the continuity of the self. Is there an ontological break, a before and after dementia self, and can the former commit the latter to decisions the former made? Can one exercise a precedent autonomy (Hertogh 2004a), that is a decision arrived at when one is considered intellectually able that substitutes when one is seen as incapable of autonomous action?

The time of one's death is also something that involves other people. Heather Davidson's poem (Box 6.3) captures the ambivalence created by contemplating loss in the context of a loved one's suffering.

Box 6.3 Good Journey

I can't remember a time
When you weren't there.
I always depended on you
And I always knew you'd care.
Now the tables have turned
And you're counting on me.
I want so much to keep you here
But I must let you go free.

At the thought that I might lose you
The spirit in me drains
But knowing if I do
For you there's no more pain.
Good journey my friend, good journey my friend
Good journey, good journey, good journey my friend.

And as I look upon your face
Expressionless your eyes
I want so much for you to stay
But I know to say, 'Goodbye'.
Thank you for your love
Now I offer love to you
And in the echo of my heart
I will forever miss you.

At the thought that I might lose you
The spirit in me drains
But knowing if I do
For you there's no more pain.
Good journey my friend, good journey my friend
Good journey, good journey, good journey my friend.

And as I reach out to touch you one last time
I'll take your hand and whisper
Good journey my friend, good journey my friend
Good journey, good journey, good journey my friend

Heather Davidson (1998) in Greenblat (2004: 87)

Conclusion

In this chapter we have examined the boundary between living and dying and the idea of the good death. We have moved between two perspectives: the social and the individual. The transition from life to death for people is managed in ways that seek to reduce the threat of death to the functioning of society. However with chronic illness, and particularly with dementia, a clear life/death boundary is elusive. People with dementia subvert many social conventions and, consequently, find themselves collectively and individually marginalized. We have considered historic and current ideas of a good death. Our focus has been on palliative care both in its reformist mode and in an observed shift towards 'good enough dying'. We have asked how some of the assumptions held in palliative care, and in chronic care more generally, can be applied to dementia. These assumptions include a belief that a good death is one that is 'chosen', or at least acknowledged and accepted by the dying person (this encapsulates an assumption of awareness and autonomy). Alternative ways of engaging with a good death have been proposed and will be further developed in our final chapter.

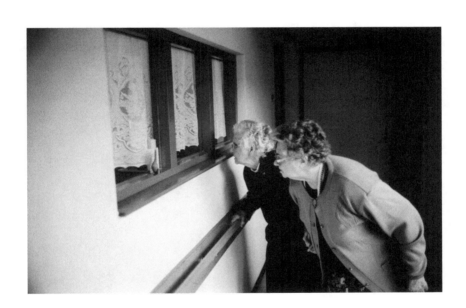

Chapter 7

Looking forward

You need the confidence here to know how to respond
to each eddy and gust ... some good friends came
alongside and gave me a tow to lunch.
Alan Kidd

Betwixt and between

The photograph that precedes this chapter shows two women looking through
a window. It is not clear if they are looking into a room from the outside or are
inside looking out. The position of the curtains in the windows indicates that
they are looking in, but the presence (and design) of the handrail on the wall
suggests they are already inside a building looking into another room. At the
very least the photograph retains an ambiguity in relation to their location. It is
a photographic image that captures the position of people with dementia both
with respect to society and also to the living–dying transition. Are they still
seen as people or does society regard them as non-persons? Are they alive or
'already dead' and hence set apart? One reading of the ambiguity of the women
in our photograph and, staying with our analogy, of people nearing the end of
their life with dementia is that they are in a liminal state. They are betwixt and
between different worlds.

The argument presented in this book has also been placed betwixt and
between different approaches to understanding care of the dying and dementia.
We followed our ambiguous cover photograph with a Sufi saying, in order to
capture our intention to draw on a considerable literature on end of life care
and another on dementia, but to also signal that we felt there was still fruitful
ground to develop when these two approaches were brought together.

We have also used the approach of differentiating between system world and
life-world concerns. This distinction has served to give some structure to the
chapters we have presented. But we have made clear throughout how each
world permeates the other. Further, we have sought to comment on experience,
and on the opportunities for change, at three interrelated levels: the level of

the individual, of the care setting and of society. A change in how we approach each of these levels has implications for all three. If the individual is viewed differently, for example approaching the self as being relational, then what follows is a clear implication that care worker's roles should include a focus on what they can do to ensure a person with dementia retains their self. The consequence would be a different staffing and training agenda, a new vision for what services could and should do and a different configuration of care. At the level of society such an approach emphasizes the continued inclusion of the person with dementia in the community and leads to what Kellehear (2005) describes as care provided *by* a community rather than care provided *for*, or *to*, an identified section of a community.

The overall argument we have made in the book has implied that a position betwixt and between can be uncomfortable but that it provides some space to develop an understanding that can draw the best aspects of different approaches together into something new and, in so doing, this can better meet the needs of people with dementia. This may feel like a messy approach. We think that in this context messy is good. There is not a single way forward or a single template we can squeeze dementia into. To seek so to do is to be trapped by the modernist paradigm that we have engaged with at various points in this book. Bauman's (1993) positive reading of postmodernity best captures the philosophical case that underlines our reluctance to settle for simple answers. Postmodernity is, he says:

> Modernity without illusions, the illusions in question boil down to the belief that the 'messiness' of the human world is but a temporary and repairable state, sooner or later to be replaced by the orderly and systematic rule of reason. The truth in question is that the 'messiness' will stay whatever we do or know, that the little orders and 'systems' we carve out in the world are brittle, until-further-notice, and as arbitrary and in the end contingent as their alternatives.

> (Bauman 1993: 32–3)

For Bauman, this change opens the possibility that we can become re-enchanted with the world, we can return dignity to emotions, indeed to all that is irrational, we can enjoy mystery, respect ambiguity and appreciate actions without purpose. To us this sounds like the sort of world where people with dementia will be better understood.[1]

Messiness accompanies dementia in the sense that:

At the system world level:

- It is incurable and, as such, troubles social assumptions about the power of reason and the optimism of progress.

---

[1] This paragraph is adapted from Small *et al.* (2006: 385–6).

In contacts with professional care services:

◆ A person may live with dementia for years. Although there are some predictable patterns of progression and some capacity to predict a likely date of death, these are not predictions that are precise enough to be easily relied on in planning services.

◆ A loss of the ability to exercise autonomy and engage in rational discussion about treatment options in people with dementia means they do not accord with prevailing orthodoxies about patient involvement and they do not fit with constructs of ageing well or the good death.

At the life-world level:

◆ The person with dementia does not exercise the rationality that allows them to conform to accepted norms of public behaviour. We have examined how this can lead to their sequestration into hidden places.

◆ An erosion of control over behaviour and over physical body functions means that places people with dementia live, and the people who care for them, are likely to have to engage with an unpredictability of temperament which can include angry and uninhibited expression and also with the messiness of the adult body.

We have argued that some of the models and assumptions concerning dementia that are currently evident in the system world, in professional orthodoxies and practice and in life-world assumptions are, themselves, part of the problem of dementia. To enhance living until you die with dementia requires understanding and seeing things differently as a precursor to doing things differently.[2]

The presence of the 'and' in the Sufi proverb at the start of the book does, as we have said above, indicate that we can look to developed literatures and examples of practice from care of the dying and dementia care to help inform our thinking about end of life care for people with dementia. However, as we have argued, both of these approaches have shortcomings. Bringing them together may be relatively simple, making them work together requires changes in each approach. If we were likening it to a marriage, the services of a matchmaker might bring two people to the altar but we need marriage guidance to help them make the marriage a success. In this concluding chapter we will think about the work that needs to be done to see care of the dying, specifically palliative care, and dementia care working together to improve end

----

2   We are grateful to Alison Kidd for helping us identify the components of our 'messy' message.

of life care. We will consider three areas. First, how can apparently opposite concepts can be reconciled? These concepts include objectivity and subjectivity, needs and rights, dying and living. Secondly, we will look at what each approach can add to the other. Finally we will return to our three levels of the individual, the care setting and society and summarize the approach we wish to support within each level and across all levels. This will return us to what has been a theme throughout the book, the relationship between the social and the self.

Attention to 'and'

In Chapter 1 we listed the 'ands' we would examine in subsequent chapters. Here we return to this list. We begin with 'living and dying', and then consider 'Care for people with dementia and care for people who are dying' although in this *and* we focus more specifically on palliative care. Our focus has also been sharpened in our return to 'life-world and system world' into a consideration of objectivity and subjectivity and in 'self and society' to a focus on needs and rights. Finally the methodological *and* we explored of discourse and narrative is now more explicitly considered in terms of what we can learn from people with dementia.

Living and dying

Considering the idea of dying alongside living with dementia involves challenging an approach taken by many people active in care provision, or in lobbying for service improvement. This approach asserts living to counter the perception prevalent at all levels, the personal, in care provision and socially, that dementia is a sort of death. But avoiding thinking about death makes it more difficult to plan for deterioration in functioning and, of course, it makes planning for death impossible. It is an approach that excludes the person at an early point in their illness, when they may still be able to play a part in advance planning, from contributing to considerations about their future, and it inhibits putting into place the changes that will maximize chances of living well until they die. It also excludes a person with dementia making a contribution to the wider discussion of dementia and the reactions of society to it. Here the example of former US President Ronald Regan's lette   the American people, following his diagnosis with Alzheimer's disease, provides a moving example of how the public understanding of dementia can be powerfully addressed by the voice of the person themselves (Box 7.1).[3]

---

[3]   It is interesting to contrast this with the secrecy that accompanied the onset of dementia in UK Prime Minister Harold Wilson 18 years before President Regan's letter (see Chapter 1).

Box 7.1 Ronald Reagan's letter to the American people

My fellow Americans:

I have recently been told that I am one of the millions of Americans who will be afflicted with Alzheimer's disease.

Upon learning this news, Nancy and I had to decide whether as private citizens we would keep this a private matter or whether we would make this news known in a public way.

In the past Nancy suffered from breast cancer and I had my cancer surgeries. We found that through our open disclosures we were able to raise public awareness. We were happy that as a result many more people underwent testing. They were treated in early stages and able to return to normal, healthy lives. So now we feel it is important to share it with you. In opening our hearts, we hope this might promote greater awareness of this condition. Perhaps it will encourage a clearer understanding of the individuals and families who are affected by it.

At the moment I feel just fine. I intend to live the remainder of the years God gives me on this earth doing the things I have always done. I will continue to share life's journey with my beloved Nancy and my family. I plan to enjoy the great outdoors and stay in touch with my friends and supporters.

Unfortunately, as Alzheimer's disease progresses, the family often bears a heavy burden. I only wish there was some way I could spare Nancy from this painful experience. When the time comes I am confident that with your help she will face it with faith and courage.

In closing let me thank you, the American people, for giving me the great honour of allowing me to serve as your president. When the Lord calls me home, whenever that may be, I will leave with the greatest love for this country of ours and eternal optimism about its future.

I now begin the journey that will lead me into the sunset of my life. I know that for America there will always be a bright dawn ahead.

Thank you, my friends. May god always bless you.

Sincerely,

Ronald Reagan

The letter appeared on November 11 1994 on the front page of virtually every newspaper in the USA and in many papers across the world. Those working in the voluntary sector in the UK report a surge of enquiries and interest immediately following the letter (personal communication).

If dying is seen as clearly demarcated from living, it is more likely that the people who may live for a long time with a terminal illness will be unsupported, and that the social barriers that are evident in the sequestration of people with dementia and of the dying will not be engaged with.

Care for people with dementia and care for people who are dying

We have contended that none of the most influential approaches that have shaped dementia care have fully engaged with dying. Palliative care, in the main, has not engaged with the needs of people with dementia. There have been exceptions developed in specific centres (although these have been primarily focused on the later stages of care) and there are national differences; overall provision in the USA is more developed than in the UK, for example. We have made the case that there is potential for integration of these two approaches and that this integration would overcome some of the limitations we have identified. We need to do more, across the whole course of dementia from diagnosis to death and beyond into bereavement care. We need to consider the individual, the organizational and the social dimensions of care and we need to be prepared to rethink some basic assumptions developed in the care of older people and in palliative care in the context of having to engage with issues of selfhood and autonomy that are not easily solved by just making minor adjustments to prevailing paradigms of care.

The contribution palliative care could make to dementia care includes technical skills and procedural practices. But palliative care's main contribution would be to reinforce the message of person-centred care in recognizing the needs of the whole person and mobilizing a multidisciplinary approach to care. Like person-centred care, at its best palliative care is optimistic and inclusive. Consultation, forward planning, and most especially an approach to care that puts the person with dementia and their experience at the centre would make a considerable difference to the many problems in end of life care discussed previously.

Similarly, there are areas of experience and insight developed in the area of general care for older people, and in dementia care, that have much to offer palliative care.

> Geriatrics stresses the importance of doing (such as ability to walk, to wash, to eat by oneself), whereas palliative care is rather focused on being. Being autonomous is to be

ruled by one's own choices, but doing and being can be combined so as to avoid both fatalism and over-treatment.

(Wary 2003: 29)

Here Wary is offering a picture of care that adds to the more philosophical engagement with being with and doing for described by Bauman that we discussed in Chapter 4 and will return to below when we consider needs and rights.

The relevant strengths within dementia care that can inform palliative care include:

- Expertise across many diseases. People with dementia live with this condition in the midst of other physical illnesses, which have to be engaged with alongside dementia. Consequently, the ability to respond to multiple pathologies is one that the palliative care world, with its characteristically single disease focus (predominantly cancer), could learn from.

- Experience in developing programmes for long-term engagement with people over many years. Individuals have access to specialist palliative care and to a hospice, in the main, for only a short period of time. As palliative care moves beyond cancer and it engages with people in the community before the terminal stage of illness there is much that can be gained from the experience of geriatrics and dementia care in terms of planning for and structuring long-term involvement with individuals, their families and the communities they live in.

- Engaging individuals who have limited or no verbal abilities and who have other cognitive impairments. Skills developed in understanding, communicating and ascertaining what preferences are and if what is provided makes a difference can be shared. Working with cognitive and behavioural changes is an area of care that hospices have tended to avoid. With cancer becoming a disease of old age, it is more likely that the people with cancer requiring palliative care are going to be living with dementia too.

There are also areas of theoretical understanding and of practice interventions developed for bereavement care that drew closely on emerging thinking in hospice and palliative care and that have been, or can be, developed to provide insights and plans for service development in dementia care. These understandings include debates about the significance of addressing (and the consequences of avoiding) the place of death in society and about the meaning of care and the importance of the self. Practice interventions have focused on the individual, family and social dimensions of loss. We have presented the detail of these developments in Chapter 3.[4]

Life-world and system world

Objectivity and subjectivity

In emphasizing subjectivity we have not wished to deny people with dementia the advantages that accrue from positivist science. The problem with the latter is not the science, it is its elevation to a position that means its proponents can deny the legitimate place of other approaches, in particular those that engage with the insights gained from subjectivity. There are advances that come from new treatments, pharmaceutical advances for example, that can and do improve the lived experience of people with dementia and their carers. While we have supported the potential that considering subjectivity brings, and specifically have argued for an engagement with narratives of peoples' lives, we also are aware that they need to be critiqued with the same rigour that we bring to a critique of the strengths and shortcomings of positivism. Both science and narrative carry with them assumptions about the possibility of exercising some sort of control. This can be over one's environment, in the case of science, and giving shape to one's life experiences through narrative. In his novel, *Scar Tissue*, Michael Ignatieff offers another possibility that does not assume that one should seek control of any sort. He examines the encounter between modernity, self-mastery and the insult of illness, and what follows if we accept biological fate:

> People like us who live by the values of self-mastery are not particularly good at dying, at submitting to biological destiny. The modern problem is not death without religious consolation, without an afterlife. The problem is that death makes the modern secular religion of self-improvement appear senseless. We are addicted to a vision of life as narrative, which we compose as we go along. In fact, we didn't have anything to do with the beginning of the story; we are merely allowed to dabble with the middle, and the end is mostly not up to us at all, but to genetics, biological fate and chance. Accepting death would mean giving up on the metaphor of life as narrative. Accepting illness would mean living ironically, accepting that we go into battle against biological fate as underdogs. We can struggle but we are likely to lose.

> (Ignatieff 1993: 68)

---

[4] We have explored the relationship between palliative care and dementia care in more detail in Small *et al.* (2006).

Ignatieff's recognition of the idea of biological fate would be familiar to people in pre-modern societies, and it may capture many people's own subjective experience when they encounter illness.

Self and society

Needs *and* rights

People nearing the end of their life, and people with cognitive impairment, have rights (see Sayers and Nesbit 2002). These may be framed positively, for example they have rights to a certain standard of care. This includes rights to adequate staffing, availability of pain relief and so on. They also have rights to be protected against things, for example against futile interventions that serve the interests of the professional but not the person nearing the end of their life. It may seem self-evident to state that people at the end of their life and with cognitive impairment have rights but, as we have argued in various parts of this book, the position is not clear. Assumptions of incapacity, of a loss of the autonomous self, of the reverence for antecedent autonomy in the form of advance directives and living wills and of the rights of others to make decisions for a person are important dimensions of the dementia environment. To safeguard rights it is necessary to ensure we meet justifiable claims for services and achieve standards of provision that are the best we can achieve. Just doing this is not sufficient. Ignatieff argues that the manner in which things are given frames another necessity.

> Rights language offers a rich vernacular for the claims an individual may make on or against the collectivity, but it is relatively impoverished as a means of expressing individuals' needs *for* the collectivity. It can only express our human ideal of fraternity as mutual respect for rights, and it can only defend the claim to be treated with dignity in terms of our common identity as rights-bearing creatures. Yet we are more than rights-bearing creatures, and there is more to respect in a person than his rights.

> (Ignatieff 1984: 13)[5]

Ignatieff's identification of the language of needs can be framed within the context of an ethics of care that draws on Bauman's 'being with' and not just 'doing for'. This is an approach that we introduced in Chapter 1 and examined in more detail in Chapter 4.

---

[5] Ignatieff explores the relationship between rights, wants and needs through a commentary on Shakespeare's *King Lear*. We have considered his insights elsewhere (see Small *et al.* 2006: 385).

Discourse and narrative: learning from people with dementia

We have argued throughout this book that the self is not diminished when there are changes in cognitive function, further that there is much that can be done to enhance the experience of living until you die with dementia. A number of ways living can be enhanced are present in people's personal accounts of living with, and caring for, someone with dementia:

- Valuing the ordinary. Lane (1998), in his account of shifting his understanding of the way his mother was dying, draws upon de Chardin (1968), who says; 'the value and interest of life is not so much to do conspicuous things ... as to do ordinary things with the perception of their enormous value' (de Chardin 1968: 156–7).

- Living in the now. Some writers have described the impact of living in the present, for example, David (cited in Noyes 2004) describes how:

    I'm robbing the reaper, I'm living at a higher rate, and we [he and his wife] can choose to have a honeymoon every night for the next hundred days! You choose in the moment. If we allow ourselves to slip into fear about the future, there's no present to find joy in. You really only connect to another person in the present. This is what you got right now and you have to make the most of it.

    (Noyes 2004: 97)

    Living in the present may be actively embraced but for others it does not solve problems, it is a consequence of illness not a life choice. Linda Grant, writing about her mother's dementia says; 'Buddhists long to move into a state beyond time, they want to rest in the moment. My mother has achieved this without any of the meditation and what state of transcendental bliss has it brought her?' (Grant 1998: 235).

- Rethinking what is important in relationships. The ability of people to relate in the ways they always had done may disappear with the progression of dementia. Other aspects of the relationship may emerge, however, as in this account presented by a daughter of her mother:

    The main point of my article, however, is to share the blessing which my mother's illness has been to me, strange as this may seem. As a child I had very little physical contact with her. She was not at all demonstrative and I longed for a mum who would sit me on her knee, cuddle me and tell me she loved me. She never did any of this – perhaps she hadn't learned how to, I don't know. What I do know is that in the past eight years, since I have had to wash her and dress her, comb her hair, help her stand up and sit down, and feed her, I have had that physical contact with her that I longed for as a child.

    Gillian Bailey, in Alzheimer's Society (2003: 12)

In a radio broadcast (Thought for the Day, BBC Radio Four, 8 February 2007) the Rev Dr Giles Fraser remembered his grandmother who had died a few days before in a nursing home. They are memories that prompt us to think that it is not only relatives like Gillian Bailey (above) who see positives in the new relationships that take shape with people with dementia. Perhaps the person themselves is not just a changed, but equally authentic self, but is also perhaps a more comfortable self.

> Most of her life she had suffered from a crushing sense of social inferiority. With Alzheimer's disease came an unforeseen sense of release ... During this time her characteristic frown slipped into a grin. And so it seems to me that right at the end of her difficult life, as she pottered about helping fellow residents and experimenting with her wardrobe, she gave some indication of the person she might have been had she found earlier release from her demons ... Perhaps that's what a rightful mind looks like. When all our plans and plotting, all our resentments and knotted histories have become foggy and indistinct, perhaps then we are released to become something like the sort of person that God has always wanted us to be.
>
> www.bbc.co.uk/religion/programmes/thought/documents/t20070208.shtml,
> downloaded 13 February 2007

Levels of change

At the individual level

Both Gillian Bailey and the Rev Dr Giles Fraser, in their recollections above, underline the importance of retaining a sense of optimism. This is consistent with our central point in relation to the individual with dementia. We have argued that the self is not destroyed or lost even if cognition is compromised. We have developed the argument elsewhere in this book that there is a focus in society (intrinsic to modernity) that emphasizes achievement in terms of acting in the world and that attributes moral worth to the manifestations of 'making oneself' (see Chapters 1 and 6 in particular). But what counts as achievement is narrowly circumscribed – many of the characteristics associated with dementia, for example impaired communication, memory loss, lack of orientation and impaired behavioural self-control, are assumed to abrogate the possibilities of achievement. The danger is that their absence is seen as negating what we have described in Chapter 4 as the moral worth of humanness because humanness is equated with action, and not with being or 'personhood'.

Jennings argues that 'Alzheimer's does not, until perhaps very, very late, close off the possibility of meaning-making activity by a person supported by the right types of interpersonal relationships and caring systems.'

He argues for the 'respect and acknowledgment of the individual as a member of the human moral community', this he calls 'moral personhood' (Jennings 2004: 275). Moral personhood is at one and the same time something that can be used to assess our reactions to people with dementia; do our actions enhance/ sustain their moral personhood or undermine it, and it can be used as a first principle that can determine the superstructures of care.

> If we come to the too-easy conclusion that Alzheimer's patients have lost moral personhood – have lost this status, this claim on our attention and response – then it will be all the easier to turn aside from these connections and all the easier to tolerate institutions and care giving systems that fail to fashion, mend, and create those connections and relationships.
>
> (Jennings 2004: 274–5)

Personhood, including moral personhood, has been engaged with as a concept and as a consequence of actions, as an underpinning input and an outcome, throughout this book. In Chapter 4 we linked a challenge to personhood with Kitwood's identification of malignant social processes and we have related these to positivism and modernity. There is now an increasing literature that engages with the way particular philosophical traditions either make the preservation of personhood in dementia more difficult or facilitate its maintenance. If personhood is intrinsically linked to the ability to recall the past and the identification of a continuity of consciousness (the position of the empiricists, epitomized by John Locke) then personhood does not survive the onset of dementia. But if personhood is located through interaction, linguistically and socially (a hermeneutic and constructivist approach), then personhood is relational and dynamic. The actions of others can enhance or diminish it (see Hughes *et al.* 2006: Post 2000b).

It is this sense of personhood as interactional and social that means we must consider the levels of the care setting and of society and not just focus on what is too easy to conceptualize as the problematic person or – at one remove from even this attribution of personhood – the problematic body that has to be hidden away, controlled and constrained.

Level of the care setting

At the level of practice innovation we have examined how a shift in approach to end of life care for people with dementia can be achieved through combining the best of existing relevant approaches. Our argument has been that this is not a simple process – when one approach *and* another are combined, as we have said, the *and* requires a reworking of each of the constituent parts.

We have also argued that any new approach has to be based on privileging subjectivity. That is, it has to be based on engaging with needs and wants from the start point of the person with dementia and building a paradigm of care from that. The psychological validity of the person with dementia's reality must be recognized and respected. We have shown that this is necessary by looking at the specific circumstances of dementia and its impact on selfhood as well as its neurological impact. To impose a regime on a person with dementia may be attractive to those who consider their technical expertise to offer the best (or only) rationale for action, people who believe they have to act 'for' and 'on behalf of' people with dementia. It will also be attractive to those people who do not see a way of accessing the views of people with dementia. Its risk is a further level of objectification that is akin to the assault on the self of the dementia syndrome.

As well as arguing about what a new approach must engage with, we have shown that a new approach is necessary by examining inadequate provision and bad practice. We have shown that a new approach is possible by presenting examples of innovative practice, including person-centred care. We have also used the comparison between the life-world and the system world as a guiding construct in this book. It has allowed us to argue for the primacy of life-world considerations, a need for the life-world to colonize the system world – in contrast to the more characteristic reverse direction of influence we see in modern societies.

At the social level

Allan Kellehear has been developing a position that argues for a health promotion and public health approach to palliative care. Both the literature he looks to, and the position he develops, resonates with our argument. For example the World Health Organization Ottawa Charter for Health Promotion (WHO 1986) recognizes the essentially social character of health and illness. 'Health care should be participatory, not something we *do to others* but a style of health care that we *do with others*' (Kellehear 2005: 25 italics in original). Living with life-threatening illness does not negate this social dynamic: one can develop health-promoting palliative care that focuses on health maintenance and the preservation of the quality of one's life even when one is living with a terminal illness (Kellehear 1999). Further, community participation can be encouraged in end of life care, a possibility Kellehear suggests is integral to the possibility of the emergence of 'Compassionate Cities' (2005).

Some steps on the journey to Compassionate Cities, through health-promoting palliative care, might include:

♦ Conceptual models to allow an understanding of living until you die. These models need to be developed in such as way that they recognize the physicality of the final stages of moving towards death. Matthews (2006) draws on Merleau-Ponty's idea of the body-subject – a person is a unity of a biological 'machine' and a consciousness. We have considered the potential contribution of Merleau-Ponty's work in Chapter 4. Our discussion of personhood and self should not ignore the quotidian reality of dying, starkly underlined for those living with the manifestations of deteriorating bodies. Conceptual models also need to capture the liminality of approaching the end of your life. That liminality is often represented by the idea of shifting one's focus from the concerns of the present world to a contemplation of one's past, or a reconciliation with one's future.

♦ Change understandings amongst clinicians about the role of medicine and the relationship between, cure, control and the maximization of quality of life, especially in ageing (Gillick 2006). In relation to dementia, underline the value of a focus on quality of life (see Chapter 5).

♦ Deprofessionalize dying via identifying it as a natural and normal stage of life, like any other (Kellehear 2005). A related argument is presented by Young and Cullen (1996), and was included in Chapter 6.

♦ Public education about dementia, ageing, dying to enhance understanding and reduce the sequestration of those nearing the end of their life.

♦ Reclaim rituals and means to support people through endings and closure in a postmodern way, that is rituals need not be imposed upon people but can grow out of the specifics of their circumstances.

We have acknowledged in Chapter 1 that our focus in this book has been on Western developed societies. All of the points made above about health promotion and public health approaches to the development of compassionate cities are of worldwide relevance. Indeed health promotion and public health can be particularly valuable approaches in countries with less developed primary, secondary and tertiary health and social care. But we must also note the facts summarized in the 2006 UN Declaration of the Rights of the Disabled (United Nations General Assembly 2006). This declaration records the worldwide agenda that emerges from a recognition that:

♦ The majority of persons with disabilities live in conditions of poverty.

♦ Peace and security are indispensable for the full protection of people with disabilities.

♦ Discrimination on any grounds including gender, race, colour, religion, language, political or other opinion, national, ethnic, indigenous or social origin, property, birth, status or age creates difficulties for people with disabilities (adapted from Annex 1 subsections p to v).

Meaningful change at the global as well as at the national level will mean engaging with these profound causes of inequality and injustice. We have argued also for the importance of considering the relationship between system and life-world concerns, and from that perspective a further level of meaningful change at the social level requires engaging with societal assumptions about the nature of the self and the centrality of cognition and autonomy. It also requires moving beyond a prevailing concern to control situations and people who threaten social order, including people with dementia and people who are dying. As we have explored in previous chapters, these societal concerns are also present at the level of professional practice. Specifically, prevailing paradigms in modern medicine are challenged by dementia. A broader perspective is required which integrates both living and dying, not just for the person with dementia, but also to reflect the particular social and cultural context that they occupy.

While this section has been structured around levels of change the central point remains that each level impacts on the others. We live, and die, within a complex of relationships both with our community, with the institutions of the state and with their representatives in the professions. These relationships can be health-preserving and promoting and they can be alienating and frighteningly destructive to our health. We are ourselves on our journey but we also journey with each other. A focus on gaining (or regaining) a sense of collective community compassion as proposed by Kellehear (2005) will provide us with at least some of the support we need.

Final thoughts

Thus we return to our journeying metaphor with which we began Chapter 2. In this chapter we have added the idea of different levels. We can use levels and journeys to help us sum up where we have got to. Throughout the book our focus has shifted from the individual to the social, from life-world to system world. We have recognized that individual agency is bounded by the socially defined parameters of what it is possible to think as well as by professional practices and policy decisions. We wish to promote an engagement with the challenge of identifying the small spaces where it is possible to devise different ways of thinking and of seeking in these to legitimize 'insider' views, the views of people with dementia and of those caring for and about them, to shape what is considered appropriate in prevailing understandings of need and in assessments of how to meet that need. Our intentions as authors have been to help open up, or further illuminate already just about open corners, to help problematize existing ways of thinking and create spaces for new ways. We have not been seeking to tear down what exists and argue for wholly new approaches. Consistent with our recognition of the potential space created by postmodernism's critique of modernism's meta-narratives, we have promoted small narratives and contingent initiatives.

Sometimes, as the last sentence above illustrates, we have presented our case using the language of social theory. We know this is not an easy language – but we are not engaged with an easy subject area and, subliminally perhaps, we have been trying to say it is vital to listen to the voices of people with dementia even when it is difficult to understand what these voices are seeking to say. You have to work harder to engage with these voices and sometimes you have to work harder with social theory, but if you want to develop critiques and plans that move beyond prevailing paradigms then ordinary ways of thinking, and ordinary language, do not always equip us to do this.

An approach that seeks to make possible the emergence of a space for change is not enough. There is also a need for the active agency of committed individuals, driven by both a critique of existing practice and a vision of what can be better. We also need to recognize, foster and heed the active agency of people with dementia, exploring in as many imaginative ways as we can how to ascertain and verify it. The active agency of people with dementia is not only difficult to interpret, it also changes as the person with dementia changes. But there is an irony evident in our desires. It is captured by Hannah, whose Grandma has dementia in Margaret Forster's novel. She knows what she wants for herself, but also knows that she may not have these desires acted on:

> When my time comes I will say I have had enough and go. That is, if my time comes like Grandma's time, if it is the same sort of time. But if it is, I won't be able to, will I?
>
> (Forster 1989: 251)

Specifically we identify the journeys that are needed:

- ◆ At the level of individual practice – from therapeutic nihilism to therapeutic optimism
- ◆ At the level of institutional care – from total institutions to therapeutic communities
- ◆ At the level of social practice – from excluding positivist and instrumental discourses to inclusive narrative

- At the level of social attitudes – from a hypercognitive society (Post 2000a) to postmodern subjectivity.
- From the colonization by the system world of the life-world to a realization that the life-world is shaping the system world.

We want the people in the photograph that preceeds this chapter to move from exclusion to engagement. We want them to be able to both look out to the world and look in to the place they live, with a sense not of anxiety but of comfort. Comfortable engagement is not a bad point on which to end.

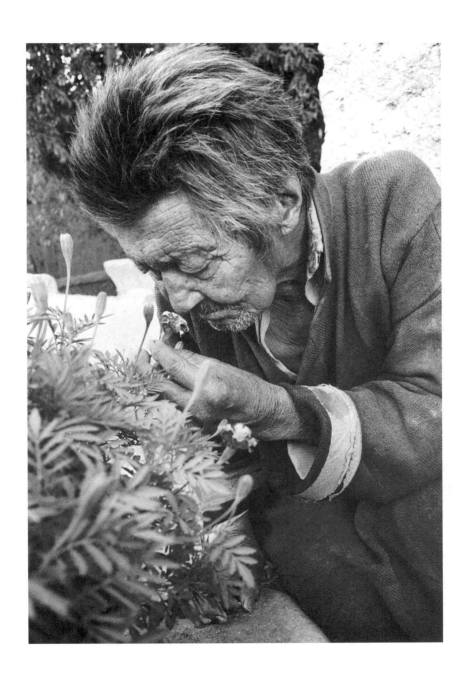

References

Aaronson NK, Bullinger M and Ahmedzai S (1988). A modular approach to quality-of-life assessment in cancer clinical trials. *Recent Results in Cancer Research*, **111**: 231–49.

Abbey J, Douglas C, Edwards H, Courtney M, Parker D and Yates P (2006). *Develop, trial and evaluate a model of multi-disciplinary palliative care for residents with end-stage dementia*. The Prince Charles Hospital Foundation, Brisbane.

Abel EK (1986). The hospice movement: institutionalizing innovation. *International Journal of Health Services*, **16**(1): 71–85.

Adams T and Clarke CL (1999). *Dementia care: developing partnerships in practice*. Ballière Tindall, London.

Addington-Hall J (1998). *Reaching out: specialist palliative care for adults with non-malignant disease*. National Council for Hospices and Specialist Palliative Care Services and Scottish Partnership Agency for Palliative and Cancer Care, London.

Addington-Hall J and Higginson I (2001). *Palliative care for non-cancer patients*. Oxford, Oxford University Press.

Agar M (1996). *The professional stranger*. Academic Press, San Diego.

Age Concern (2002). *End of life issues*. Policy Unit. Age Concern England, London.

Agich GJ (1993). *Autonomy and long-term care*. Oxford University Press, Oxford.

Ahronheim JC, Morrison RS, Baskin SA, Morris J and Meier DE (1996). Treatment of the dying in the acute care hospital – advanced dementia and metastatic cancer. *Archives of Internal Medicine*, **156**(18): 2094–100.

Ahronheim JC, Morrison S and Morris J (2000). Palliative care in advanced dementia: A ramdomized controlled trial and descriptive analysis. *Journal of Palliative Medicine*, **3**(3): 265–73.

Alaszewski A and Manthorpe J (1993). Quality and the welfare services: A literature review. *British Journal of Social Work*, **23**(6): 653–65.

Albert SM and Logsdon RG (2000). *Assessing quality of life in Alzheimer's disease*. Springer Publishing, New York.

Albinsson L and Strang P (2003a). Differences in supporting families of dementia patients and cancer patients: A palliative perspective. *Palliative Medicine*, **17**(4): 359–67.

Albinsson L and Strang P (2003b). Existential concerns of families of late-stage dementia patients: Questions of freedom, choices, isolation, death, and meaning. *Journal of Palliative Medicine*, **6**(2): 225–35.

Alzheimer Europe (2005). Advance directives: a position paper. Available at www.alzheimer-europe.org, accessed 13 November 2006.

Alzheimer's Society (2003). *In memory of memories*. London, Alzheimer's Society.

Alzheimer's Society (2007a). UK's first emergency appeal to challenge NICE. Available at http://www.alzheimers.org.uk/News_and_Campaigns/News/060207nice.htm. Accessed 16 February 2007.

Alzheimer's Society (2007b). Position statement: decision making. Available at http://www.alzheimers.org.uk/News_and_Campaigns/Policy, accessed 16 February 2007.

Alzheimer's Society (2006). Policy positions: demography. Available at www.alzheimers. org.uk/News_and_Campaigns/Policy_Watch/demography.htm. Accessed 15 March 2006.

American Academy of Paediatrics (2000). Palliative care for children. *Paediatrics*, **106**(2): 351–7.

Aneshensel C, Pearlin L, Mullan J and Zarit S (1995). *Profiles in caregiving: The unexpected career*. Academic Press Inc., London.

Antonovsky A (1979). *Health, stress and coping*. Jossey-Bass, San Fransisco.

Antonovsky A (1987). *Unravelling the mystery of health: How people manage stress and stay well*. Jossey-Bass, San Fransisco.

Applebaum R (2001). Foreword. In LS Noelker and Z Harel (eds.). *Linking quality of long term care and quality of life*, pp. ix–xi. Springer Publishing Company, New York.

Appleyard B (2007). *How to live forever or die trying: On the new immortality*. Simon and Schuster, London.

Arie T (1970). The first year of the Goodmayes psychiatric service for old people. *Lancet*, **ii**: 1179–82.

Arie T (1977). Issues in the psychiatric care of older people. In AN Exton-Smith and J Grimley Evans (eds.). *Care of the elderly*. Academic Press, New York.

Arie T and Isaacs AD (1977). The development of psychiatric services in Britain. In AD Isaacs and F Post (eds.). *Studies in geriatric psychiatry*, pp. 241–261. John Wiley, Chichester.

Arie T and Jolley D (1982). Making services work: organisation and style of psychogeriatric services. In R Levy and F Post (eds.). *The psychiatry of late life*, pp. 222–51. Blackwell, Oxford.

Ariès P (1974). *Western attitudes toward death: From the Middle Ages to the present*. Johns Hopkins University, Baltimore.

Ariès P (1981). *The hour of our death*. Knopf, New York.

Ariès P (1985). *Images of man and death*. Cambridge, MA, Harvard University Press.

Ariss S, Grant E, Downs M, Fernandez B, Gallagher R, Cherry D and Barclay M (2006). Piloting a consumer-directed intervention to improve primary care for dementia in the UK. *Dementia: the International Journal of Social Research and Practice*, **5**(3): 456–62.

Armstrong D (1987). Silence and truth in death and dying. *Social Science and Medicine*, **24**(8): 651–7.

Audit Commission (2000). *Forget me not: Mental health services for older people*. Audit Commission, London. Available at http://www.audit-commission.gov.uk.

Australian Government Department of Health and Ageing (2004). *Guidelines for a palliative approach in residential aged care*. Canberra, Rural Health and Palliative Care Branch, Australian Government Department of Health and Ageing.

Australian Institute of Health and Welfare (1998). *Australia's health 1998: the sixth biennial health report of the Australian Institute of Health and Welfare*. AIHW, Canberra.

Baldwin C (2005). Narrative ethics and people with severe mental illness. *Australian and New Zealand Journal of Psychiatry*, 39, 11–12; 1022–1029.

Baldwin C (2006a). Narrative, ethics and ethical narratives in dementia. In A Burns and B Winblad (eds.). *Severe Dementia*, pp. 215–26. John Wiley and Sons, Chichester.

Baldwin C (2006b). Making difficult decisions at the end of life. In J Hughes (ed.). *Palliative care in severe dementia*, pp. 97–104. Quay Books, London.

Baldwin C and Capstick A (2007 forthcoming). *A Tom Kitwood reader: dementia theory and practice*. Open University Press, Buckingham.

Baldwin R and Murray M (eds.). (2003). *Younger people with dementia: a multidisciplinary approach*. Martin Dunitz, London.

Baldwin R, Chaplin R, Murray M and Kindell J (2003). Assessment and referral. In R Baldwin and M Murray (eds.). *Younger people with dementia: a multidisciplinary approach*, pp. 43–57. Martin Dunitz, London.

Ballard C (2000). Criteria for the diagnosis of dementia. In J O'Brien, D Ames and A Burns (eds.). *Dementia*, 2nd edn, pp. 29–40. Arnold, London.

Ballard C, Fossey J, Chithramohan R, Howard R, Burns A, Thompson P, Tadros G and Fairbairn A (2001a). Quality of care in private sector and NHS facilities for people with dementia: Cross-sectional survey. *BMJ*, **323**(7310): 426–7.

Ballard C, O'Brien J, James I, Mynt P, Lana M, Potkins D, Reichelt K, Lee L. Swann A and Fossey J (2001b). Quality of life for people with dementia living in residential and nursing home care. *International Psychogeriatrics*, **13**(1): 93–106.

Ballenger JF (2006). *Self, senility, and Alzheimer's disease in modern America: A history*. Johns Hopkins University Press, Baltimore.

Banerjee S (2007). *Specialist health services for people with dementia – development and delivery of care*. Report to the Alzheimer's Society. Alzheimer's Society, London.

Barnes I and Thomandl S (2004). Coma care in end-stage dementia. *Canadian Nursing Home* **15**(1): 50–51.

Bartlett R, O'Connor D (2007). From personhood to citizenship: Broadening the lens for dementia practice and research. *Journal of Ageing Studies*, **21**(2): 107–118.

Bauman Z (1992). *Mortality, immortality and other life strategies*. Polity Press, Oxford.

Bauman Z (1993). *Postmodern ethics*. Blackwell, Oxford.

Bayer A (2006). Death with dementia – the need for better care. *Age and Ageing*, **35**(1): 101–2.

Bayley J (1998). *Iris: A memoir of Iris Murdoch*. Duckworth, London.

Beattie ERA, Algase DL and Song J (2004). Behavioural symptoms of dementia: their measurement and intervention. *Ageing and Mental Health*, **8**(2): 109–16.

Beauchamp TL and Childress JF (1994). *Principles of biomedical ethics*. Oxford University Press, Oxford.

Bender M (2003). *Explorations in dementia: theoretical and research studies into the experience of remediable and enduring cognitive losses*. Jessica Kingsley, London.

Bender M, Haddow L, Hartley T and Wainwright T (2002). Do charities have to devalue their clients to get donations? *Journal of Dementia Care*, 10, (4) 36–37.

Bennett A (2005). *Untold stories*. Faber and Faber, London.

Berger PL and Luckmann T (1967). *The social construction of reality*. Penguin, Harmondsworth.

Berrios G (2000). Dementia: historical overview. In J O'Brien, D Ames and A Burns (eds.). *Dementia*, 2nd edn, pp. 1–13. Arnold, London.

Bertman SL (1991). *Facing death: Images, insights and interventions: a handbook for educators, healthcare professionals, and counsellors*. Hemisphere, New York.

Bird M (2000). Psychosocial management of behavioural problems in dementia. In J O'Brien, D Ames and A Burns (eds.). *Dementia*, 2nd edn, pp. 603–13. Arnold, London.

Birren JE and Deutchman DE (1991) Concepts and content of quality of life in the later years: An overview. In M Lawton (ed.). *A multidimensional view of quality of life in frail elders*, pp. 344–60. Academic Press, San Diego.

Black D and Jolley D (1990). Slow euthanasia? The deaths of psychogeriatric patients. *BMJ* **300**(6735): 1321–3.

Bloch M and Parry J (1982). *Death and the regeneration of life*. Cambridge University Press, Cambridge.

Boden C (1998). *Who will I be when I die?* Harper Collins, Melbourne.

Bogdan R and Taylor SJ (1989) Relationships with severely disabled people: the social construction of humaneness. *Social Problems*, **36**(2): 135–48.

Bond J (1999). Quality of life for people with dementia: Approaches to the challenge of measurement. *Ageing and Society*, **19**(5): 561–79.

Bowes A and Wilkinson H (2003). 'We didn't know it would get that bad': South Asian experiences of dementia and service response. *Health and Social Care in the Community*, **11**(5): 387–96.

Bowling A (1995). What things are important thing in people's lives? A survey of the public's judgements to inform scales of health-related quality of life. *Social Science and Medicine*, special issue on 'Quality of life'. **10**: 1447–62.

Bowling A (1997). *Measuring health: A review of quality of life measurement scales*. Open University Press, Buckingham.

Brechling BG and Kuhn D (1989). A specialized hospice for dementia patients and their families. *The American Journal of Hospice Care*, **6**(3): 27–30.

Brenner PR (1998). The experience of Jacob Perlow Hospice: Hospice care of patients with Alzheimer's disease. In L Volicer and A Hurley (eds.). *Hospice care for patients with advanced progressive dementia*, pp. 257–75. Springer Publishing, New York.

Brod M, Stewart AL, Sands L and Walton P (1999a). Conceptualization and measurement of quality of life in dementia: the Dementia Quality of Life instrument (DQoL). *The Gerontologist*, **39**(1): 25–35.

Brod MI, Stewart AL and Sands L (1999b). Conceptualisation of quality of life in dementia. *Journal of Mental Health and Ageing*, **5**: 7–19.

Brodaty H and Low L-F (2005). Involvement of carers, consumers and the broader community. In Draper B, Melding P and Brodaty H (eds.). *Psychogeriatric service delivery: An international perspective*, pp. 293–308. Oxford University Press, Oxford.

Brody H (1994). My story is broken: can you help me fix it? *LitMed*, **13**: 91–4.

Brooker D (1995). Looking at them looking at me: A review of observational studies into the quality of institutional care for elderly people with dementia. *Journal of Mental Health and Ageing*, **4**(2): 145–56.

Brooker D (2004). What is person-centred care for people with dementia? *Reviews in Clinical Gerontology*, **13**: 212–22.

Brooker D (2005). Dementia Care Mapping: A review of the research literature. *The Gerontologist*, **45**(Special Issue 1): 11–18.

Brooker D (2007). *Person-centred dementia care: making services better*. Jessica Kingsley Publishers, London.

Brookmeyer R, Corrada MM, Curriero FC and Kawas C. (2002). Survival following a diagnosis of Alzheimer disease. *Archives of Neurology*, **59**(11): 1764–7.

Brown University (2005). *TIME: Toolkit of instruments to measure end-of-life care*. Available at http://www.chcr.brown.edu/pcdc/Quality.htm (downloaded 14 December 2005).

Bruce E (1998). Holding on to the story: older people, narrative, and dementia. In G Roberts and J Holmes (eds.). *Healing stories*, pp. 181–205. Oxford University Press, Oxford.

Bruce E, Surr C and Tibbs MA (2002). *A special kind of care: improving well-being in people living with dementia*. MHA Care Group, Derby.

Bryden C (2005). *Dancing with dementia*. Jessica Kingsley, London.

Buber M (1970). *I and thou*. Clark, Edinburgh (first published in German in 1923).

Burns A (2001). *Textbook of geriatric neuropsychiatry*, 2nd edn, book review. *British Journal of Geriatric Psychiatry*, **179**: 185.

Burns A (ed.) (2005). *Standards in dementia care*. Taylor and Francis, London.

Burns A and Winblad B (2006). *Severe dementia*. Wiley and Sons, London.

Burns AR, Jacoby R, Luthert P and Levy R (1990). Cause of death in Alzheimer's disease. *Age and Ageing*, **19**(5): 341–4.

Bury M (1982). Chronic illness as biographical disruption. *Sociology of Health and Illness*, **4**: 167–82.

Byock IR and Merriman MP (1998). Measuring quality of life for patients with terminal illness: The Missoula-VITAS quality of life index. *Palliative Medicine*, **12**(4): 231–44.

Calkins MP (2001). The physical and social environment of the person with Alzheimer's disease. *Aging and Mental Health*, **5**(Suppl 1): 126–30.

Calman K (1984). Quality of life in cancer patients – an hypothesis. *Journal of Medical Ethics*, **10**(3): 124–7.

Cancer Relief Macmillan Fund (1994). *Organisational audit for specialist palliative care services*. Cancer Relief Macmillan Fund, London.

Cantley C (2005). Dementia services development centres in the UK. In A Burns (ed.). *Standards in dementia care*, pp. 287–93. Taylor and Francis, London.

Cantley C, Woodhouse J and Smith M (2005). *Listen to us: involving people with dementia in planning and developing services*, Dementia North, Northumbria University, Newcastle upon Tyne.

Caracciolo F (2006). *Alzheimer: a journey together*. Jessica Kingsley, London.

Cassell CK (2004). Foreword. In RB Purtillo and HAMJ ten Have (eds.). *Ethical foundations of palliative care for Alzheimer's disease*, pp. ix–xi. Johns Hopkins University Press, London.

Chalfont G (2007). *Design for nature and dementia*. Jessica Kingsley, London.

Chalfont GE (2005). Creating enabling outdoor environments for residents. *Nursing and Residential Care*, **7**: 454–7.

Chassin MR, Galvin RW and the National Roundtable on Health Care Quality (1998). The urgent need to improve health care quality: Institute of medicine national roundtable on health care quality. *Journal of the American Medical Association*, **280**(11): 1000–05.

Chaudhury H (1999). Self and reminiscence of place: a conceptual study. *Journal of Aging and Identity*, **4**(4): 231–54.

Chaudhury H (2002). Place-biosketch as a tool in caring for residents with dementia. *Alzheimer's Care Quarterly*, **3**(1): 42–5.

Chekov A (1917). *The cherry orchard*. Scribners, New York.

Cheston R and Bender M (1999). *Understanding dementia. The man with the worried eyes.* Jessica Kingsley, London.

Cheston R (1998). Psychotherapeutic work with people with dementia: a review of the literature. *British Journal of Medical Psychology,* **71**(3): 211–31.

Clare L (2002b). Developing awareness about awareness in early-stage dementia. *Dementia,* **1**: 295–312.

Clare L (2002a). We'll fight it as long as we can: coping with the onset of Alzheimer's disease. *Ageing and Mental Health,* **6**: 139–48.

Clare L (2003). Managing threats to self: Awareness in early-stage Alzheimer's disease. *Social Science and Medicine,* **57**: 1017–29.

Clark D (1998). Originating a movement: Cicely Saunders and the development of St Christopher's Hospice, 1957–1967. *Mortality* **3**(1): 43–63.

Clark D (1999). Cradled to the grave? Preconditions for the hospice movement in the UK, 1948–67. *Mortality,* **4**: 225–47.

Clark D (2000). Palliative care history: a ritual process. *European Journal of Palliative Care* **7**(2): 50–55.

Clark D (2002). Between hope and acceptance: The medicalisation of dying. *BMJ,* **324**(7350): 905–7.

Clark D and Seymour J (1999). *Reflections on palliative care.* Open University Press, Buckingham.

Clark D, Small N, Wright M, Winslow M and Hughes N (2005). *A bit of heaven for the few? An oral history of the modern hospice movement in the United Kingdom.* Observatory Press, Lancaster.

Clarke A, Hanson E J and Ross H (2003). Seeing the person behind the patient: enhancing the care of older people using a biographical approach. *Journal of Clinical Nursing,* **12**(5): 697–706.

Clarke C (1999). Family care-giving for people with dementia: some implications for policy and professional practice. *Journal of Advanced Nursing,* **29**(3): 712–20.

Clarke R (2004). Precious experiences beyond words. *Journal of Dementia Care,* **12**(3): 22–3.

Clinch JJ, Dudgeon D and Schipper H (1998). Quality of life assessment in palliative care. In D Doyle, GWC Hanks and N MacDonald (eds.). *Oxford textbook of palliative medicine,* pp. 83–94. Oxford University Press, Oxford.

Cohan M (1997). Stages of dementia: An overview. In CR Kovach (ed.). *Late-stage dementia care: A basic guide,* pp. 3–11. Taylor and Francis, Washington, DC.

Cohen C (1983). 'Quality of life' and the analogy with the Nazis. *Journal of Medicine and Philosophy,* **8**(2): 113–35.

Cohen D and Eisdorfer C (1986). *The loss of self: a family resource for the care of Alzheimer's Disease and associated disorders.* WW Norton and Company, London.

Cohen E (2003). *The house on Beartown Road.* Random House, New York.

Cohen SR, Mount BM, Strobel MG and Bui F (1995). The McGill Quality of Life Questionnaire: A measure of quality of life appropriate for people with advanced disease. A preliminary study of validity and acceptability. *Palliative Medicine,* **9**: 207–19.

Cohen-Mansfield J and Lipson S (2002). Pain in cognitively impaired nursing home residents: how well are physicians diagnosing it? *Journal of the American Geriatrics Society,* **50**(6): 1039–44.

Cohen-Mansfield J and Werner P (1997). Management of verbally disruptive behaviors in nursing home residents. *J Gerontol A Biol Sci Med Sci*, **52**: M369–77.

Collins C, Liken M, King S and Kokonakis C (1993). Loss and grief among family caregivers of relatives with dementia. *Qualitative Health Research*, **3**(2): 236–53.

Collopy BJ (1988). Autonomy in long term care: some crucial distinctions. *Gerontolgoist*, **28**(Suppl): 10–17.

Cooke R (2006). The Amis papers. *The Observer Review*, Oct 1st: pp 8–9.

Corr C (1993). Death in a modern society. In D Doyle, GWC Hanks and N Macdonald (eds.). *The Oxford Textbook of Palliative Medicine*, pp. 28–36. Oxford Medical Publications, Oxford.

Corr C and Corr D (1983). *Hospice care: principles and practice*. Faber and Faber, London.

Corr C, Corr KM and Ramsey S (2004). Alzheimer's disease and the challenge for hospice. In K Doka (ed.). *Living with grief Alzheimer's disease*, pp. 227–44. Hospice Foundation of America, Washington, DC.

Cotrell V and Schulz R (1993). The perspective of the patient with Alzheimer's disease: a neglected dimension of dementia research. *The Gerontologist*, **33**(2): 205–211.

Cox S and Cook A (2002). Caring for people with dementia at the end of life. In J Hockley and D Clark (eds.). *Palliative care for older people in care homes*, pp. 86–103. Open University Press, Buckingham.

Cox S and Keady J (1998). *Younger people with dementia: planning, practice and development*. Jessica Kingsley, London.

Craib I (1992). *Modern social theory*. St Martin's Press, New York.

Darton R, Netten A and Forder J (2003). The cost implications of the changing population and characteristics of care homes. *International Journal of Geriatric Psychiatry*, **18**(3): 236–43.

Davies E and Higginson I (2004). *Better palliative care for older people*. World Health Organisation, Copenhagen.

Davies S and Nolan M (2003). 'Making the best of things': relatives' experiences of decisions about care-home entry. *Ageing and Society*, **23**(4): 429–50.

Davis R (1989). *My journey with Alzheimer's disease*. Tyndale House, Wheaton, Il.

de Chardin TP (1968). *Letters to two friends, 1926–1952*. New American Library, New York.

de Vries K (2003). Palliative care for people with dementia. In T Adams and J Manthorpe (eds.). *Dementia care*, pp. 114–35. Arnold, London.

de Vries K (in press). Matters of the heart: the CMHN and palliative care. In J Keady, C Clarke and S Page (eds.). *Partnerships in community mental health nursing and dementia care*. Open University Press, Buckingham.

de Vries K, Sque M, Bryan K, and Abu-Saad H (2003). Variant Creutzfeldt-Jakob disease: need for mental health and palliative care team collaboration. *International Journal of Palliative Nursing*, **9**(12): 512–20.

Dean R, Proudfoot R and Lindesay J (1993). The Quality of Interactions Schedule (QUIS): Development, reliability and use in the evaluation of two Domus units. *International Journal of Geriatric Psychiatry*, **8**(10): 819–26.

Dekkers WJM (2004). Autonomy and the lived body in cases of severe dementia. In RB Purtillo and HAMJ ten Have (eds.). *Ethical foundations of palliative care for Alzheimer's disease*. pp. 115–30. Johns Hopkins University Press, London.

Denzin NK (1992). *Symbolic interactionism and cultural studies: the politics of interpretation.* Blackwell, Oxford.

Denzin NK (1997). *Interpretive ethnography: ethnographic practices for the 21st century.* Sage, London.

Department of Health (1989). *Working for patients.* CM555, HMSO, London.

Department of Health (1992). *The Patients' Charter for England.* Department of Health, London.

Department of Health (1997). *The new NHS: modern dependable.* Department of Health, London.

Department of Health (2000). *The NHS cancer plan. A plan for investment. A plan for reform.* Department of Health, London.

Department of Health (2001a). *National service framework for older people.* Department of Health, London.

Department of Health (2001b). *Involving patients and the public in healthcare: A discussion document.* Department of Health, London.

Department of Health (2005). *Commissioning a patient-led NHS.* Retrieved August 2006 from www.dh.gov.uk/assetRoot/04/11/67/17/04116717.pdf.

Department of Health (2006a). *Our health, our care, our say: A new direction for community services.* White Paper. Department of Health, London.

Department of Health (2006b). *A new ambition for old age: next steps in implementing the national service framework for older people.* Department of Health, London.

Diamond M C (2001). Enrichment, response of the brain. *Encyclopedia of Neuroscience,* 3rd edition, Elsevier Science, Amsterdam.

Doka KJ (ed.) (1989). *Disenfranchised grief: recognizing hidden sorrow.* Lexington Books, Lexington, MA.

Doka KJ (ed.) (2004). *Living with grief: Alzheimer's disease.* Hospice Foundation of America, Washington, DC.

Doka KJ and Aber R (2002). Psychological loss and grief. In K Doka (ed.). *Disenfranchised grief: new directions, challenges and strategies for practice,* Research Press, Champaign, IL.

Donabedian A (1980). *Explorations in quality assessment and monitoring.* Health Administration Press, Ann Arbour, MI.

Donabedian A (1988). Quality assessment and assurance: Unity of purpose, diversity of means. *Inquiry,* 25(1): 173–92.

Dorenlot P and Fremontier M (eds) (2006). *Supporting and caring for people with dementia throughout end of life.* Fondation Mederic Alzheimer, Paris.

Downs M (1997). The emergence of the person in dementia research. *Ageing and Society,* 17(5): 597–607.

Downs M (2000). Dementia in a social and cultural context: an idea whose time has come. *Ageing and Society,* 20: 369–75.

Downs M (2005). Awareness and dementia: in the eye of the beholder. *Ageing and Mental Health,* 9: 381–3.

Downs M, Brooker D and Bruce E (2005). The practice of person-centred dementia care in the UK. In A Burns (ed.). *Standards in dementia care,* pp. 13–19. Taylor and Francis, London.

Downs M, Small N and Froggatt K (2006c). Person-centred care for people with severe dementia. In A Burns and B Winblad (eds.). *Severe dementia*, pp. 193–204. London: Wiley and Sons.

Downs M, Small N and Froggatt N (2006b). Explanatory models of dementia: links to end-of-life care. *International Journal of Palliative Nursing*, **12**(5): 209–213.

Downs M, Turner S, Bryans M, Wilcock J, Keady J, Levin E, O'Carroll R, Howie K and Iliffe S (2006a). Effectiveness of educational interventions in improving detection and management of dementia in primary care: a cluster randomized controlled study. *BMJ*, **332**: 692–6.

Doyal L and Gough G (1991). *A theory of human need*. Macmillan, Basingstoke.

Draper B, Melding P and Brodaty H (2005). *Psychogeriatric service delivery: an international perspective*. Oxford University Press, Oxford.

Drickamer MA and Lachs MS (1992). Should patients with Alzheimer's disease be told their diagnosis? *New England Journal of Medicine*, **326**: 947–51.

Edelman P, Fulton BR and Kuhn D (2004). Comparison of dementia specific quality of life measures in adult day centres. *Home Health Care Services Quarterly*, **23**(1): 25–42.

Eliot TS (1988). *East Coker. The four quartets*. Harcourt Brace and Company, San Diego. (First published 1944)

Embleton Tudor, L (2004). *The person-centred approach: a contemporary introduction*. Palgrave Macmillan, Basingstoke.

Engedal K (2005). Norwegian Centre for dementia research, service development and education. In A Burns (ed.). *Standards in dementia care*, pp. 295–301. Taylor and Francis, London.

Engel GL (1977). The need for a medical model: a challenge for biomedicine. *Science*, **196**: 129–36.

Enthovan A (1985). *Reflections on the management of the NHS*. Nuffield Provincial Hospitals Trust, London.

Erkinjuntti T (2000). Vascular dementia: an overview. In J O'Brien, D Ames and A Burns (eds.). *Dementia*, 2nd edn, pp. 623–34. Arnold, London.

Evers H (1993). The development of geriatric medicine. In J Johnson and R Slater (eds.). *Ageing and later life*, pp. 319–26. Sage, London.

Evers MM, Purohit D, Perl D, Khan K and Marin DB (2002). Palliative and aggressive end-of-life care for patients with dementia. *Psychiatric Services*, **53**(5): 609–13.

Evers MM, Meier DE (2002). Assessing differences in care needs and service utilisation in geriatric palliative care patients. *Journal of Pain and Symptom Management*, **23**(5): 424–432.

Expert Advisory Group on Cancer (1995). *A policy framework for commissioning cancer services: a report by the Expert Advisory Group on Cancer to the Chief Medical Officers of England and Wales*. Department of Health and Welsh Office, London.

Exton-Smith AN and Evans GJ (eds) (1977). *Care of the elderly*. Academic Press, New York.

Faulkner W (2000). *As I lay dying*. New York, The Modern Library. Originally published by Random House in 1930.

Feil N (1982). *Validation: the Feil method*. Edward Feil Productions, Cleveland, Ohio.

Feinberg LF and Whitlatch CJ (2001). Are persons with cognitive impairment able to state consistent choices? *The Gerontologist*, **41**: 374–82.

Ferri CP, Prince M, Brayne C, Brodaty H, Fratiglioni L, Gnaguli M, Hall K, Hasegawa H, Huang Y, Jorm A, Mathers C, Menezes PR, Rimmer E and Scazufca M (2005). Global prevalence of dementia: a Delphi consensus study. *The Lancet*, **366**(9503): 2112–17.

Field D and Addington-Hall J (1999). Extending specialist palliative care to all? *Social Science and Medicine*, **48**(9): 1271–80.

Finkel SI, Costa e Silva J, Cohen G, Miller S and Sartorius N (1996). Behavioural and psychological signs and symptoms of dementia: a consensus statement on current knowledge and implications for research and treatment. *International Psychogeriatrics*, **8**(Suppl 3): 497–500.

Finnema E (2000). *Emotion-oriented care in dementia: a psychosocial approach*. Vrije Universiteit, Amsterdam.

Forbes S, Bern-Klug M and Gessert C (2000). End-of-life decision making for nursing home residents with dementia. *Image: Journal of Nursing Scholarship*, **32**(3): 251–8.

Formiga F, Olmeod C, Soto AL and Pujol R (2004). Dying in hospital of severe dementia: palliative decision-making analysis. *Aging Clinical and Experimental Research*, **16**(5): 420–1.

Forster M (1989). *Have the men had enough?* Penguin Books, London.

Forstl H (2000). What is Alzheimer's disease? In J O'Brien, D Ames and A Burns (eds.). *Dementia*, 2nd edn, pp. 371–82. Arnold, London.

Fortinsky RH (2001). Health care triads and dementia care: integrative framework and future directions. *Aging and Mental Health*, 5(Suppl 1): S35–S48.

Fossey J, Ballard C, Juszczak E, James I, Alder N, Jacoby R and Howard R (2007). Effect of enhanced psychosocial care on antipsychotic use in nursing home residents with severe dementia: cluster randomised trial. *BMJ*, **332**: 756–61.

Foucault M (1967). *Madness and civilization*. Tavistock, London.

Foucault M (1972). *The archaeology of knowledge and the discourse on language*. Pantheon Books, New York.

Fox P (1989). From senility to Alzheimer's disease: the rise of the Alzheimer's disease movement. *Millbank Quarterly*, **67**(1): 58–102.

Fox P (2000). The role of the concept of Alzheimer's disease in the development of the Alzheimer's Association in the United States. In PJ Whitehouse, K Maurer and JF Ballenger (eds.). *Concepts of Alzheimer's disease: Biological, clinical and cultural perspectives*, pp. 209–33. The Johns Hopkins University Press, London.

Friedell M (2000). Potential for rehabilitation in Alzheimer's disease. Available at http://members.aol.com/MorrisFF/Rehab.html, accessed 13 February 2007.

Friedell M (2002). Awareness: a personal memoir on the changing quality of life in Alzheimer's. *Dementia: the International Journal of Social Research and Practice*, 1: 359–66.

Friedell M (2003). Dementia survival: a new vision. *Alzheimer's Care Quarterly*, **4**(2): 79–84.

Froggatt A (1988). Self-awareness in early dementia. In B Gearing, M Johnson and T Heller (eds.). *Mental health problems in old age: a reader*, pp. 131–8. John Wiley and Sons, Chichester.

Froggatt K (2001). Life and death in English nursing homes: sequestration or transition? *Ageing and Society*, **21**: 319–32.

Froggatt K (2005). 'Choice over care at the end of life'. Implications of the End of Life Initiative for older people in care homes. *Journal of Research in Nursing*, **10**(2): 189–202.

Froggatt KA (2004). *Palliative care in care homes for older people*. The National Council for Palliative Care, London.

Froggatt KA, Downs M and Small N (in press). Palliative care for people with dementia: principles, practice and implications. In R Woods and L Clare (eds.). *Handbook of the clinical psychology of ageing*, 2nd edn. Chichester: Wiley

Fulton RL and Bendikson R (1994). *Death and identity*, 3rd edn. Philadelphia: Charles Press.

Garfinkel H (1967). *Studies in ethnomethodology*. Prentice-Hall, Englewood Cliffs, NJ.

Gass TE (2004). *Nobody's home: candid reflections of a nursing home aide*. Cornell University Press, Ithaca, New York.

Gelber RD, Goldhirsch A and Cole BF (1993). Evaluation of effectiveness: Q-TwiST. The International Breast Cancer Study Group. *Cancer Treatment Reviews*, **19**(Suppl A): 73–84.

Gibson MC, Bol N, Woodbury MG, Beaton C and Janke C (1999). Comparison of caregivers', residents', and community-dwelling spouses' opinions about expressing sexuality in the institutional setting. *Journal of Gerontological Nursing*, **25**(4): 30–9.

Giles L, Cameron I and Crotty M (2003). Disability in older Australians: projections for 2006–13. *Medical Journal of Australia*, **179**(3): 130–3.

Giles S (1993). Depth charges. *Health Service Journal*, 18 Nov: 15.

Gillick M (2006). *The denial of aging*. Harvard University Press, Cambridge, MA.

Gillick MR (2000). Rethinking the role of tube feeding in patients with advanced dementia. *The New England Journal of Medicine*, **342**(3): 206–10.

Gilligan C (1982). *In a different voice*. Harvard University Press, Cambridge.

Gjerdingen DK, Neff JA, Wang M and Chaloner K (1999). Older persons' opinions about life-sustaining procedures in the face of dementia. *Archives of Family Medicine*, **8**(5): 421–5.

Glaser B and Strauss A (1965). *Awareness of dying*. Aldine, Chicago.

Glaser BG and Strauss AL (1968). *Time for dying*. Aldine, Chicago.

Glass AP (1991). Nursing home quality: A framework for analysis. *Journal of Applied Gerontology*, **10**(1): 5–18.

Godlove C, Sutcliffe C, Bagley H, Cordingley L, Challis D, Huxley P and Burns A (2004). *Towards quality care: outcomes for older people in care homes*. Ashgate, Aldershot.

Goffman E (1959). *The presentation of self in everyday life*. Pelican Books, London.

Goldsmith M (2004). *In a strange land. People with dementia and the local church*. 4M Publications, Southwell.

Good P and Stafford B (2001). Inpatient palliative care is evidence based. *Palliative Medicine*, **15**(6): 493–8.

Gorer G (1955). The pornography of death. *Encounter*, **5**: 49–52.

Gorer, G. (1965). *Death, grief and mourning*. Doubleday, Garden City, NY.

Graham N, Lindesay J, Katona C, Bertolote JM *et al.* (2003). Reducing stigma and discrimination against older people with mental disorders: a technical consensus statement. *International Journal of Geriatric Psychiatry*, **18**: 670–8.

Graneheim UH, Norberg A and Jansson L (2001). Interaction relating to privacy, identity, autonomy and security: an observational study focussing on a woman with dementia and 'behavioural disturbances', and on her care providers. *Journal of Advanced Nursing*, **36**(2): 256–65.

Grant L (1998). *Remind me who I am, again*. Granta Books, London.

Grayling AC (2005). Right to die. *BMJ*, **330**: 799.

Greenblat C (2004). *Alive with Alzheimer's*. University of Chicago Press, Chicago.

Greenhalgh T and Hurwitz B (1999). Narrative-based medicine: Why study narrative? *BMJ*, **318**: 48–50.

Gubrium J (1986). *Oldtimers and Alzheimer's: the descriptive organisation of senility*. JAI Press Inc., London.

Gubrium JF (2000). Narrative practices and the inner worlds of the Alzheimer disease experience. In PJ Whitehouse, M Konrad and JF Ballenger (eds.). *Concepts of Alzheimer disease: Biological, clinical and cultural perspectives*, pp. 181–204. The John Hopkins University Press, Baltimore.

Habermas J (1975). *Legitimation crisis*. Beacon Press, Boston, MA.

Habermas J (1979). *Communication and the evolution of society*. Beacon Press, Boston, MA.

Habermas J (1984). *The theory of communicative action: reason and the rationalisation of society*. Beacon Press, Boston, MA.

Habermas J (1987). *The theory of communicative action. Lifeworld and system: a critique of functionalist reason*. Beacon Press, Boston, MA.

Halling E (2004). Still here, wherever here is. In KJ Doka (ed.). *Living with grief: Alzheimer's disease*, pp. 127–34. Hospice Foundation of America, Washington.

Hancock K, Chang E, Johnson A, Harrison K, Daly J, Easterbrook S, Noel M, Luhr-Taylor M and Davidson P (2006). Palliative care for people with dementia. *Alzheimer's Care Quarterly*, **7**(1): 49–57.

Hanrahan P and Luchins DJ (1995). Access to hospice programs in end-stage dementia: A national survey of hospice programs. *Journal of the American Geriatric Society*, **43**(1): 56–9.

Hanrahan P, Raymond M, McGowan E and Luchins DJ (1999). Criteria for enrolling dementia patients in hospice: a replication. *The American Journal of Hospice and Palliative Care*, **16**(1): 395–400.

Harman G and Clare L (2006). Illness representations and lived experience in early-stage dementia. *Qualitative Health Research*, **16**: 484–502.

Harris PB (2002). *The Persons with Alzheimer's Disease: Pathways to Understanding the Experience*. Johns Hopkins University Press, London.

Harrison S and Mort M (1998). Which champions, which people? Public and user involvement in health care. *Soc. Policy and Admin*, **32**: 60–70.

Harrison S, Hunter D, Marnoch G and Pollitt C (1989). *The impact of general management in the NHS*. Open University Press, Milton Keynes.

Harrison T (1993). *Black daisies for the bride*. Faber and Faber, London.

Hart B, Sainsbury P and Short S (1998). Whose dying? A sociological critique of the 'good death'. *Mortality*, **3**(1): 65–77.

Health Advisory Service (1998). *Not because they are old: an independent inquiry into the care of older people in acute settings in general hospitals*. Pavilion Publishing, Brighton.

Heidrich SM and Ryff CD (1993). Physical and mental health in later life: the self-system as mediator. *Psychology and Ageing*, **8**(3): 327–38.

Hepburn KW, Caron W, Luptak M, Ostwald S, Grant L and Keenan JM (1997). The family stories workshop: stories for those who can't remember. *The Gerontologist*, **37**(6): 827–32.

Herbert LP, Scherr J, Benias D, Bennett DA and Evans D (2003). Alzheimer's disease in the US population: prevalence estimates using the 2000 census. *Archives of Neurology*, **60**: 1119–22.

Hermans D, Lisaerde J and Triau E (1989). Sense and non-sense of a technological health care model in terminally ill demented patients. The first international conference on the palliative care of the elderly. *Journal of Palliative Care*, **5**(4): 39–42.

Herskovitz E (1995). Struggling over subjectivity: debates about the 'self' and Alzheimer's disease. *Medical Anthropology Quarterly*, **9**(2): 146–64.

Hertogh C (2004a). Autonomy, competence and advanced directives: the physician proposes, the patient disposes? In GMM Jones and BML Miesen (eds.). *Care-giving in dementia*, 3, pp. 391–403. Hove, Brunner-Routledge.

Hertogh C (2004b). Between autonomy and security: Ethical questions in the care of elderly persons with dementia in nursing homes. In GMM Jones and BML Miesen (eds.). *Care-giving in dementia*, 3, pp. 375–90. Brunner-Routledge, Hove.

Higginson I (1998). *Clinical and organizational audit in palliative care*. In D Doyle, GWC Hanks and N MacDonald (eds.). *Oxford Textbook of Palliative Medicine*, pp. 67–81. Oxford University Press, Oxford.

Higginson I and McCarthy M (1993). Validity of the support team assessment schedule: Do staff ratings reflect those made by patients or their families? *Palliative Medicine*, **8**(4): 282–90.

Hilton C (2005). The clinical psychiatry of late life in Britain from 1950 to 1970: an overview. *International Journal of Geriatric Psychiatry*, **20**: 423–8.

Hirakawa Y, Masuda Y, Kuzuya M, Kimata T, Iguchi A and Uemura K (2006). End-of-life experience of demented elderly patients at home: findings from DEATH Project. *Psychogeriatrics*, **6**: 60–7.

HM Government (2005). *Mental Capacity Act*. The Stationery Office, London.

Hockey J (1990). *Experiences of death. An anthropological account*. Edinburgh University Press, Edinburgh.

Hockey J and James A (1993). *Growing up and growing old: ageing and dependency in the life course*. Sage, London.

Hofland B (1994). When capacity fades and autonomy is constricted: a client-centred approach to residential care. *Generations*, **18**(4): 31–5.

Hoggart R (2006). *Promises to keep: thoughts in old age*. Continuum, London.

Holden RT and Woods RT (1995). *Positive approaches to dementia care*. Edinburgh: Churchill Livingstone.

Holst G and Hallberg IR (2003). Exploring the meaning of everyday life, for those suffering from dementia. *American Journal of Alzheimer's Disease and Other Dementias*, **18**(6): 359–65.

Holstein M and Cole TR (1996). Reflections on age, meaning and chronic illness. *Journal of Ageing and Identity*, **1**(1): 7–22.

Hope T (1994). Personal identity and psychiatric illness. In, A Phillips Griffiths, (ed.). *Philosophy, psychology and psychiatry*, pp 131–43, Cambridge University Press, Cambridge.

Hospice Information Service (2006). *The directory of hospice and specialist palliative care services*. Help the Hospices, London.

House of Commons Health Committee (2004). *Palliative care fourth report of session 2003–04*. House of Commons, London.

Howard R, Ballard C, O'Brien J and Burns A (2001). Guidelines for the management of agitation in dementia. *International Journal of Geriatric Psychiatry*, **16**: 714–17.

Hughes J (2004). The practice and philosophy of palliative care in dementia. *Nursing and Residential Care*, **6**(1): 27–30.

Hughes JC (2001). Views of the person with dementia. *Journal of Medical Ethics*, **27**: 86–91.

Hughes JC (2003). Quality of life in dementia: an ethical and philosophical perspective. *Expert Review of Pharmacoeconomics and Outcomes Research*, **3**(5): 525–34.

Hughes JC (ed). (2005). *Palliative care in severe dementia*. Quay Books, London.

Hughes JC and Baldwin C (2006). *Ethical issues in dementia care: making difficult decisions*. Jessica Kingsley, London.

Hughes JC, Louw SJ and Sabat SR (eds) (2006). *Dementia: mind, meaning and the person*. Oxford University Press, Oxford.

Hughes JC, Robinson L and Volicer L (2005). Specialist palliative care in dementia. *BMJ*, **330**(7482): 57–8.

Humphreys SC (1981). Death and time. Mortality and immortality. In SC Humphreys and H King (eds.). *The anthropology and archaeology of death*, pp. 261–83. Academic Press, London.

Hunter D (1993). Rationing and health gain. *Critical Public Health*, **4**(1): 27–32.

Ignatieff M (1984). *The needs of strangers*. Chatto and Windus, London.

Ignatieff M (1993). *Scar tissue*. Chatto and Windus, London.

Illich I (1976). *Limits to medicine: medical nemesis. The expropriation of health*. Marion Boyars, London.

Illich I (1995). Pathogenesis, immunity, and the quality of public health. *Qualitative Health Research*, **5**(1): 7–14.

Innes A (2002). The social and political context of formal dementia care provision. *Ageing and Society*, **22**(4): 483–99.

James N and Field D (1992). The routinization of hospice: charisma and bureaucratization. *Social Science and Medicine*, **12**(3): 1363–75.

Jefferys M (2000). Recollections of the pioneers of the geriatric medicine specialty. In J Bornat, R Perks, P Thompson and J Walmsley (eds.). *Oral history, health and welfare*, pp. 75–97. Routledge, London.

Jennings B (2000). A life greater than the sum of its sensations: ethics, dementia and the quality of life. In SM Albert and RG Logsdon (eds.). *Assessing quality of life in Alzheimer's disease*, pp. 169–70. Springer Publishing, New York.

Jennings B (2004). Alzheimer's disease and the quality of life. In KJ Doka (ed.). *Living with grief: Alzheimer's disease*, pp. 247–58. Hospice Foundation of America, Washington.

Jett KF (2006). Mind-loss in the African American community: dementia as a normal part of aging. *Journal of Aging Studies*, **20**(1): 1–10.

Jolley D and Baxter D (1997). Life expectation in organic brain disease. *Advances in Psychiatric Treatment*, **3**: 211–18.

Jolley DJ and Arie T (1978). Organisation of psychogeriatric services. *British Journal of Psychiatry*, **132**: 1–11.

Jones G (1992). Introduction. In Jones G.M.M. and Miesen B.M.L. (eds.). *Care-giving in dementia*, volume **1**: Routledge, London: 1–4.

Kabcenell A and Roessner J (2002). Pursuing perfection. *Journal of Quality Improvement*, **28**(5): 268–78.

Kalish RA (1966). A continuum of subjectively perceived death. *The Gerontologist*, **6**(2): 73–6.

Kastenbaum R (1995). *Death, society and human experience*, 5th edn. Allyn and Bacon, Boston, MA.

Katz J, Sidell M and Komaromy C (2000). Death in homes: bereavement needs of relatives and staff. *International Journal of Palliative Nursing*, **6**(6): 274–9.

Kayser-Jones J (2002). The experience of dying: an ethnographic nursing home study. *The Gerontologist*, **42**(Special Issue III): 11–19.

Kayser-Jones J, Schell E, Lyons W, Kris AE, Chan J and Beard RL (2003). Factors that influence end-of-life care in nursing homes: The physical environment, inadequate staffing, and lack of supervision. *The Gerontologist*, **43**(Special Issue II): 76–84.

Keady J and Gilliard J (2002). Testing times: the experience of neuropsychological assessment for people with suspected Alzheimer's disease. In P Harris (ed.). *The person with Alzheimer's disease: pathways to understanding the experience*, pp. 3–28. John Hopkins University Press, London.

Keady J and Nolan M (1994). Younger onset dementia: developing a longitudinal model as the basis for a research agenda and as a guide to interventions with sufferers and carers. *Journal of Advanced Nursing*, **19**(4): 659–69.

Keady J, Clarke C and Adams T (2003). *Community mental health nursing and dementia care: practice perspectives*. Open University Press, Maidenhead.

Keady J, Clarke C and Page S (eds) (in press). *Partnerships in community mental health nursing and dementia care*. McGraw-Hill, London.

Keady, J and Keady, J (2005). The wrong shoes; living with memory loss. *Nursing Older People*, **17**(9): 36–7.

Kearney M (1992). Palliative medicine – just another specialty? *Palliative Medicine*, **6**: 39–46.

Keene J, Hope T, Fairburn CG and Jacoby R (2001). Death and dementia. *International Journal of Geriatric Psychiatry*, **16**(10): 969–74.

Kellehear A (1999). *Health promoting palliative care*. Oxford University Press, Oxford.

Kellehear A (2005). *Compassionate cities: public health and end-of-life care*. Routledge, London.

Kfir N and Slevin M (1991). *Challenging cancer – from chaos to control*. Tavistock/Routledge, London.

Kihlgren M, Hallgren A, Norberg A, Karlsson I (1994). Integrity promoting care of demented patients: patterns of interaction during morning care. *International Journal of Ageing and Human Development*, **39**(4): 303–19.

Killick J and Allan K (2001). *Communication in the care of people with dementia*. Open University Press, Buckingham.

Killick J and Allan K (2006). *The Good Sunset project*. Hammond Care Group, Sydney.

Killick J and Cordonnier C (2000). *Openings*. Hawker Publications, London.

Kissell JL (2004). The moral self as patient. In RB Purtilo and HAMJ ten Have (eds.). *Ethical foundations of palliative care for Alzheimer's disease*, pp. 131–45. John Hopkins University Press, London.

Kitwood T (1987). Explaining senile dementia: the limits of neuropathological research. *Free Associations*, **10**: 117–40.

Kitwood T (1990). The dialectics of dementia: with particular reference to Alzheimer's disease. *Ageing and Society*, **10**(2): 177–96.

Kitwood T (1993). Person and process in dementia. *International Journal of Geriatric Psychiatry*, **8**(7): 541–5.

Kitwood T (1993). Towards a theory of dementia care: the interpersonal process. *Ageing and Society*, **13**(1): 51–67.

Kitwood T (1994). The concept of personhood and its implications for the care of those who have dementia. In G Jones and B Miesen (eds.). *Caregiving in dementia*, volume 2, pp. 3–13. Routledge, London.

Kitwood T (1995). Positive long-term changes in dementia: some preliminary observations. *Journal of Mental Health*, **4**(2): 133–44.

Kitwood T (1996). A dialectical framework for dementia. In RT Woods (ed.). *Handbook of the clinical psychology of ageing*. pp. 267–282. John Wiley and Sons, London.

Kitwood T (1997a). *Dementia reconsidered, the person comes first*. Open University Press, Maidenhead.

Kitwood T (1997b). The experience of dementia. *Aging and Mental Health*, **1**(1): 13–22.

Kitwood T (1998). Toward a theory of dementia care: ethics and interaction. *The Journal of Clinical Ethics*, **9**(1): 23–34.

Kitwood T and Benson S (eds) (1995). *The new culture of dementia care*. Hawker Publications, London.

Kitwood T and Bredin K (1992a). A new approach to the evaluation of dementia care. *Journal of Advances in Health and Nursing Care*, **1**(5): 41–60.

Kitwood T and Bredin K (1992b). Towards a theory of dementia care: personhood and well-being. *Ageing and Society*, **12**(3): 269–87.

Kitwood T and Bredin K (1993). *Evaluating dementia care: the DCM method*. Bradford Dementia Research Group, University of Bradford.

Klass D, Silverman PR and Nickman SL (1996). *Continuing bonds: new understandings of grief*. Taylor and Francis, Washington, DC.

Klein R (1989). *The politics of the NHS*, 2nd edn. Longman, London.

Kleinman A (1995). *Writing at the margin: discourse between anthropology and medicine*. University of California Press, Berkeley.

Kontos PC (2004). Ethnographic reflections on selfhood, embodiment and Alzheimer's disease. *Ageing and Society*, **24**: 829–49.

Kovach CR (1997). Maintaining personhood: philosophy, goals, program development and staff education. In CR Kovach (ed.). *Late stage dementia care: a basic guide*, pp. 25–43. Taylor and Francis, London

Kübler-Ross E (1969). *On death and dying*. Routledge, London.

Kuhn D, Ortigara A and Farran C (1997). A continuum of care in Alzheimer's disease. *Adv Prac Nurs Q*, **2**(4): 15–21.

Lamberg JL, Person CJ, Kiely DK and Mitchell SL (2005). Decisions to hospitalize nursing home residents dying with advanced dementia. *Journal of American Geriatrics Society*, **53**(8): 1396–401.

Lamerton R (1980). *Care of the dying*. Penguin, Harmondsworth.

Lane B (1998). *The solace of fierce landscapes: exploring desert and mountain spirituality*. Oxford University Press, New York.

Lawton J (2000). *The dying process: patients' experiences of palliative care*. Routledge, London.

Lawton M (1991). A multidimensional view of quality of life in frail elders. In J Birren, J Lubben, J Rowe and D Deutchman (eds.). *The concept and measurement of quality of life in the frail elderly*, pp. 3–27. Academic Press, San Diego.

Lawton MP (1997). Quality of life in Alzheimer's disease research. *Alzheimer's Disease and Associated Disorders*, **11**(Suppl 6): 91–9.

Lawton MP, Moss M, Hoffman C, Grant R, Have TT and Kleban MH (1999). Health, valuation of life, and the wish to live. *The Gerontologist*, **39**(4): 406–16.

Levenson R (2004). Lessons from the end of life. *BMJ*, **329**(7476): 1244.

Lewin A (2004). *Watching the kingfisher*. Inspire, Peterborough.

Lidz CW, Fischer L and Arnold RM (1992). *The erosion of autonomy in long-term care*. University Press, New York.

Lindesay J, Marudkar M, van Diepen E and Wilcock G (2002) The second Leicester survey of memory clinics in the British Isles. *International Journal of Geriatric Psychiatry*, **17**(1): 41–7.

Lloyd-Williams M (1996). An audit of palliative care in dementia. *European Journal of Cancer Care*, **5**(1): 53–5.

Lloyd-Williams M and Payne S (2002). Can multidisciplinary guidelines improve the palliation of symptoms in the terminal phase of dementia? *International Journal of Palliative Nursing*, **8**(8): 370–5.

Luchins DJ and Hanrahan P (1993). What is appropriate health care for end-stage dementia? *Journal of American Geriatric Society*, **41**(1): 25–30.

Lyman KA (1989). Bringing the social back in: a critique of the biomedicalization of dementia. *The Gerontologist*, **29**(5): 597–605.

Lyman KA (1998). Living with Alzheimer's disease: the creation of meaning among persons with dementia. *Journal of Clinical Ethics*, **9**(1): 49–57.

Lyotard F (1984). *The postmodern condition: a report on knowledge*. University of Manchester Press, Manchester.

MacDonald A and Cooper B (2007). Long-term care and dementia services: an impending crisis. *Age and Ageing*, **36**: 16–22.

Mackenzie J (2006). Stigma and dementia: East European and South Asian family carers negotiating stigma in the UK. *Dementia: the International Journal of Social Research and Practice*, **5**(2): 233–47.

MacLaverty B (2005). The assessment. In O Frawley (ed.). *New Dubliners*, pp. 61–78. New Island, Dublin.

MacQuarrie CR (2005). Experiences of early stage Alzheimer's disease: understanding the paradox of acceptance and denial. *Ageing and Mental Health*, **9**(5): 430–41.

Madan TN (1992). Dying with dignity. *Social Science and Medicine*, **4**: 425–32.

Magaziner J, German P, Zimmerman SI, Hebel JR, Burton L, Gruber-Baldini AL, May C and Kittner S (2000). The prevalence of dementia in a statewide sample of new nursing home admissions aged 65 and older: diagnosis by expert panel. *The Gerontologist*, **40**(6): 663–72.

Maguire C, Kirby M, Coen R, Lawlor B, Coakley D and O'Neill D (1996) Family members' attitudes toward telling the patient with Alzheimer's Disease their diagnosis. *BMJ*, **313**: 529–30.

Margallo-Lana M, Swann A, O'Brien J, Fairbairn A, Reichelt K, Potkins D, Mynt P and Ballard C (2001). Prevalence and pharmacological management of behavioural and psychological symptoms amongst dementia sufferers living in care environments. *International Journal of Geriatric Psychiatry*, **16**: 39–44.

Marie Curie Memorial Foundation (1952). *Report on a national survey concerning patients nursed at home*. Marie Curie Memorial Foundation, London.

Marriott A (2003). Helping families cope with dementia. In T Adams and J Manthorpe (eds.). *Dementia care*, pp. 187–201. Arnold, London.

Marshall M (2000). *Homely: the guiding principle of design for dementia*. In J O'Brien, D Ames and A Burns (eds.). *Dementia*, pp. 233–9. Arnold, London.

Marshall M (ed.) (2005). *Perspectives on rehabilitation and dementia*. Jessica Kingsley Publishers, London.

Marshall M and Tibbs MA (2006). *Social work and people with demenitia*. Policy Press Bristol.

Matthews E (2006). Dementia and the identity of the person. In, JC Hughes, SJ Louw and S Sabat (eds.). *Dementia. Mind, meaning and the person*, pp. 163–177. Oxford University Press, Oxford.

McCarthy M, Addington-Hall J and Altmann D (1997). The experience of dying with dementia: a retrospective study. *International Journal of Geriatric Psychiatry*, **12**(3): 404–9.

McCormack B (2001). Negotiating partnerships with older people. *Ageing and Society*, **21**: 417–46.

McCubbin HI, Thompson EA and Fromer JE (1998). *Stress, coping and health in families: sense of coherence and resiliency*. Sage, Thousand Oaks, CA.

McGough R (1983). *The Mersey sound*, revised edn. Penguin, Harmandsworth, Middlesex.

McGowin D (1994). *Living in the labyrinth. A personal journey through the maze of Alzheimer's*. Delacorte Press, New York.

McGrath AM and Jackson GA (1996). Survey of prescribing in residents of nursing homes in Glasgow. *BMJ*, **314**: 611–12.

McKeith I (2000). Dementia with Lewy bodies: a clinical overview. In, J O'Brien, D Ames and A Burns (eds.). *Dementia*, 2nd edn, pp. 685–97. Arnold, London.

McNamara B (2004). Good enough death: autonomy and choice in Australia palliative care. *Social Science and Medicine*, **58**(5): 929–38.

McNamara B, Waddell C and Colvin M (1994). The institutionalisation of the good death. *Social Science and Medicine*, **39**(11): 1501–8.

McNeil BJ, Weichselbaum R and Pauker SG (1981). Speech and survival: tradeoffs between quality and quantity of life in laryngeal cancer. *New England Journal of Medicine*, **305**(17): 982–7.

Mead GH (1932). *Mind, self and society from the standpoint of a social behaviourist*, (edited by Charles W. Morris). University of Chicago, Chicago.

Mellor PA and Shilling C (1993). Modernity, self-identity and the sequestration of death. *Sociology*, **27**: 411–31.

Merleau-Ponty M (1962). *The phenomenology of perception*. London, Routledge and Kegan Paul.

Michel JP, Pautex S, Zekry D, Zulian G and Gold G (2002). End-of-life care of persons with dementia. *Journal of Gerontology Medical Sciences*, **57A**(10): M640–M644.

Miesen BML (1992). Attachment theory and dementia. In GMM Jones and BML Miesen (eds.). *Care-giving in dementia*, volume 1, pp. 38–56. London, Routledge.

Miesen BML and Jones GMM (eds) (2006). *Care-giving in dementia*, volume 4. London, Routledge.

Mirea A and Cummings J (2000). Neuropsychiatric aspects of dementia. In J O'Brien, D Ames and A Burns (eds.). *Dementia*, 2nd edn, pp. 61–79. Arnold, London.

Mitchell SL, Kiely DK and Hamel MB (2004). Dying with advanced dementia in the nursing home. *Archives of Internal Medicine*, **164**(3): 321–6.

Mitchell SL, Teno, JM, Miller SC and Mor V (2005). A national study of the location of death for older persons with dementia. *Journal of the American Geriatrics Society*, **53**(2): 299–305.

Moller DW (1990). *On death without dignity. The human impact of technological dying*. Baywood Publishing Company, Amityville, NY.

Moniz-Cook E and Woods RT (1997). The role of memory clinics and psychosocial intervention in the early stages of dementia. *International Journal of Geriatric Psychiatry*, **12**: 1143–5.

Moniz-Cook E, Manthorpe J, Carr I, Gibson G and Vernooij-Dassen M (2006). Facing the future: a qualitative study of older people referred to a memory clinic prior to assessment and diagnosis. *Dementia: the International Journal of Social Research and Practice*, **4**(3): 442–9.

Moody HR (1988). From informed consent to negotiated consent. *The Gerontologist*, **28**(3 Suppl): 64–70.

Moskowitz EH and Nelson JL (1995). The best laid plans. *Hastings Center Report*, **25**(6 Suppl): 53–5.

Mozley C, Huxley P, Sutcliffe C, Bagley H, Burns A, Challis D and Cordingley L (1999). Not knowing where I am doesn't mean I don't know what I like: cognitive impairment and quality of life responses in elderly people. *International Journal of Geriatric Psychiatry*, **14**(9): 776–83.

Mulkay M (1993). Social death in Britain. In D Clark (ed.). *The sociology of death*, pp. 31–49. Blackwell, Oxford.

Mulkay M and Ernst J (1991). The changing profile of social death. *Arch Europ Sociol*, **XXXII**(4): 172–96.

Murphy E (2000). Epilogue. In J O'Brien, D Ames and A Burns (eds.). *Dementia*, 2nd edn, pp. 917–19. Arnold, London.

National Council for Hospice and Specialist Palliative Care Services and Scottish Partnership Agency (2000). *Positive partnerships. Occasional paper 17*. NCHSPC, London.

National Council for Hospices and Specialist Palliative Care Services. (1995). *Occasional paper 8, Specialist palliative care: a statement of definitions*. NCHSPC, London.

National Council for Palliative Care (2006). *Exploring palliative care for people with dementia.* National Council for Palliative Care, London.

National Institute for Clinical Excellence (2004). *Guidance on cancer services. Improving supportive and palliative care for people with cancer.* National Institute for Clinical Excellence, London.

National Institute for Health and Clinical Excellence and Social Care Institute for Clinical Excellence (2006). *Dementia; supporting people with dementia and their carers in health and social care.* Clinical Guideline CG42. NICE/SCIE, London.

Neale R, Brayne C and Johnson AL (2001). Cognition and survival: an exploration in a large multicentre study of the population aged 65 years and over. *International Journal of Epidemiology*, **30**(6): 1383–8.

Neary D (2000). Frontotemporal dementia. In J O'Brien, D Ames and A Burns (eds.). *Dementia*, 2nd edn, pp. 737–46. Arnold, London.

Noddings N (1984). *Caring. A feminine approach to ethics and moral education.* University of California Press, Berkeley.

Noddings N (2002). *Starting at home. Caring and social policy.* University of California Press, Berkeley.

Noelker LS and Harel Z (2001). *Linking quality of long-term care and quality of life.* Springer Publishing, New York.

Nolan M, Grant G and Keady J (1996). *Understanding family care: a multi-dimensional model of caring and coping.* Open University Press, Buckingham.

Nolan MR, Davies S and Grant G (eds) (2001). *Working with older people and their families.* Open University Press, Buckingham.

Nolan MR, Davies S, Brown J, Keady J and Nolan M (2004). Beyond 'person-centred' care: a new vision for gerontological nursing. *International Journal of Older People Nursing*, **13**(3a): 45–53.

Norberg A (1998). Interaction with people suffering from severe dementia. In A Wimo, B Jonsson, G Karlsson and B Wingblad (eds.). *Health economics of dementia*, pp. 113–21. John Wiley and Sons, Chichester.

Norberg A (2001). Communication in the care of people with severe dementia. In HML Nussbaum and JF Nussbaum (eds.). *Ageing, communication and health: linking research and practice for successful ageing*, pp. 157–73. Lawrence Erlbaum Associates, New Jersey.

Notter J, Spijker T and Stomp K (2004). Taking the community into the home. *Health and Social Care in the Community*, **12**(5): 448–53.

Noyes L (2004). Journeys into Alzheimer's. In K Doka (ed.). *Living with grief: Alzheimer's disease*, pp. 87–98. Hospice Foundation of America, Washington, DC.

Nuland S (1997). *How we die.* Vintage, London.

Nussbaum M (2004). Care, dependency and social justice: a challenge to conventional ideas of the social contract. In P Lloyd-Sherlcok (ed.). *Living longer: ageing, development and social protection*, pp. 275–9. Zed Books, London.

O'Boyle C, McGee A, Hickey K, Joyce C and O'Malley K (1993). *Schedule for the Evaluation of Individual Quality of Life (SEIQoL): a direct weighting procedure for Quality of Life domans (SEIQoL-DW). Administration Manual.* Royal College of Surgeons, Dublin.

O'Boyle CA, McGee H, Hickey A, O'Malley K and Joyce CRB (1992). Individual quality of life in patients undergoing hip replacement. *The Lancet*, **339**: 1088–91.

Oliver C (1999). Ordering the disorderly. *Education and Ageing*, **14**(2): 171–85.

Olson, E (2003). Dementia and neurodegenerative diseases. In RS Morrison and DE Meier (ed.). *Geriatric palliative care*. pp. 160–72. Oxford University Press, Oxford.

OPCS (1985). *Mortality statistics, 1841–1980*. Series DH1 No. 15, HMSO, London.

Owen JE, Goode KT and Haley WE (2001). End of life care and reactions to death in African-American and white family caregivers of relatives with Alzheimer's disease. *Omega: The Journal of Death and Dying*, **43**(4): 349–61.

Parfit D (1984). *Reasons and persons*. Clarendon Press, Oxford.

Parker-Oliver D, Porock D and Zweig S (2004). End-of-life care in U.S. nursing homes: a review of the evidence. *Journal of American Medical Directors Association*, **5**(3): 147–55.

Paterniti DA (2003). Claiming identity in a nursing home. In JF Gubrium and JA Holstein (eds.). *Ways of aging*, pp. 58–74, Blackwell, Oxford.

Payne S, Hillier R, Langley-Evans A and Roberts T (1996). Impact of witnessing death on hospice patients. *Social Science and Medicine*, **43**(12): 1785–94.

Payne S, Kerr C, Hawker S, Seamark D, Davis C, Roberts H, Jarrett N, Roderick P and Smith H (2004). Community hospitals: an under-recognized resource for palliative care. *J R Soc Med*, **97**: 428–31.

Peace D (2006). *The damned united*. Faber and Faber, London.

Perri 6 and Peck E (2004). New Labour's modernisation of the public sector: a neo-Durkheimian approach and the case of mental health services. *Public Administration*, **82**(1): 83–108.

Perrin, T and May, H (1999). *Wellbeing in dementia: an occupational approach for therapists and carers*. Churchill Livingstone, London.

Pettit B (2000). The role of primary care in the management of dementia. In, J O'Brien, D Ames and A Burns (eds.). *Dementia*. Second edition, pp. 242 – 249. Arnold, London.

Pfeffer N and Coote A (1991). *Is quality good for you?* Institute for Public Policy Research, Social Policy Paper 5, London.

Phinney A (2002). Living with the symptoms of Alzheimer's disease. In PB Harris (ed.). *The person with Alzheimer's disease: pathways to understanding the experience*, pp. 49–74. The Johns Hopkins University Press. Baltimore, MD.

Phinney A and Chesla CA (2003). The lived body in dementia. *Journal of Aging Studies*, **17**(3): 283–99.

Phipps AJ and O'Brien JT (2002). Memory clinics and clinical governance – a UK perspective. *International Journal of Geriatric Psychiatry*, **17**: 1128–32.

Pinner G and Bouman WP (2003). Attitudes of patients with mild dementia and their carers towards disclosure of the diagnosis. *International Psychogeriatrics*, **15**: 279–88.

Pirsig RM (1974). *Zen and the art of motorcycle maintenance*. William Morrow and Company, New York.

Pitt B (1974). *Psychogeriatrics: an introduction to the psychiatry of old age*. Churchill Livingstone, London.

Plummer K (2001). *Documents of life 2: an invitation to critical humanism*. Sage, London.

Porell F (2005). Discretionary hospitalization of nursing home residents with and without Alzheimer's disease. *Journal of Aging and Health*, **17**(2): 207–38.

Post SG (2000a). The concept of Alzheimer disease in a hypercognitive society. In PJ Whitehouse, K Maurer and JF Ballenger (eds.). *Concepts of Alzheimer disease*, pp. 245–56. Johns Hopkins University Press, Baltimore.

Post SG (2000b). *The moral challenge of Alzheimer disease: ethical issues from diagnosis to dying*. Johns Hopkins University Press, Baltimore.

Potkins D, Bradley S, Shrimanker J, O'Brien J, Swann A and Ballard C (2000). End of life treatment decisions in people with dementia: carers' views and the factors which influence them. *International Journal of Geriatric Psychiatry*, **15**: 1005–8.

Pratt R and Wilkinson H (2003). A psychosocial model of understanding the experience of receiving a diagnosis of dementia. *Dementia*, **2**(2): 181–99.

Pullman P (2001). *The amber spyglass*. Scholastic Press, Southam, Warwickshire.

Rabins PV, Kasper JD, Kleinman L, Black BS and Patrick DL (1999). Concepts and methods in the development of the ADRQL: an instrument for assessing health-related quality of life in persons with Alzheimer's disease. *Journal of Mental Health Aging*, **5**(1): 33–48.

Rader J, Doan J and Schwab M (1985). How to decrease wandering, a form of agenda behaviour. *Geriatric Nursing*, **6**(4): 196–9.

Rando TA (1986). *Parental loss of a child*. Research Press, Champaign, IL.

Rando TA (2000). *The six dimensions of anticipatory mourning*. In TA Rando (ed.). Clinical dimensions of anticipatory mourning: theory and practice in working with the dying, their loved ones, and their caregivers, pp. 51–101. Research Press, Champaign, IL.

Raushi TM (2004). Something was not right. In K Doka (ed.). *Living with grief: Alzheimer's disease*, pp. 99–109. Hospice Foundation of America, Washington.

Rawls J (1972). *A Theory of Justice*. Oxford University Press, Oxford.

Reisberg B (1988). Functional Assessment Staging (FAST). *Psychopharm Bulletin*, **24**: 653–9.

Rich BA (1998). Personhood, patienthood, and clinical practice: reassessing advance directives. *Psychology, Public Policy, and Law*, **4**(3): 610–28.

Robinson L, Clare L and Evans K (2005a). Making sense of dementia and adjusting to loss: psychological reactions to a diagnosis of dementia in couples. *Ageing and Mental Health*, **9**(4): 337–47.

Robinson L, Hughes J, Daley S, Keady J, Ballard C and Volicer L (2005b). End-of-life care and dementia. *Reviews in Clinical Gerontology*, **15**: 135–48.

Rogers CR (1961). *On becoming a person*. Houghton Mifflin, Boston.

Rosenhan D (1973). On being sane in insane places. *Science*, **179**: 250–8.

Rosser RM (1985). A history of the development of health indices. In GT Smith (ed.). *Measuring the social benefits of medicine*, Office of Health Economics, London.

Roth M (1955). The natural history of mental disorder in old age. *Journal of Mental Science*, **101**(423): 281–301.

Rovner BW, Steele C, Shmuely DS and Folstein MF (1996). A randomised trial of dementia care in nursing homes. *J Am Geriatr Soc*, **44**: 7–13.

Rundell J (1991). Jurgen Habermas. In P Beilharz (ed.). *Social theory*, Allen and Unwin, Sydney. 133–40.

Sabat S (1991a). Facilitating conversation via indirect repair: a case study of Alzheimer's disease. *The Georgetown Journal of Languages and Linguistics*, **2**(3–4): 284–96.

Sabat SR (1991b). Turn-taking, turn giving and Alzheimer's disease: a case study of conversation. *The Georgetown Journal of Languages and Linguistics*, **2**(2): 167–81.

Sabat SR (2001). *The experience of Alzheimer's disease: life through a tangled veil*. Blackwell Publishers, Malden, MA.

Sabat SR (2005). Capacity for decision-making in Alzheimer's disease: selfhood, positioning and semiotic people. *Australian and New Zealand Journal of Psychiatry*, **39**(11–12): 1030–35.

Sabat SR (2006a). Implicit memory and people with Alzheimer's disease: implication for caregiving. *American Journal of Alzheimer's Disease and Other Dementias*, **21**(1): 11–14.

Sabat SR (2006b). Mind, meaning and personhood in dementia: the effects of positioning. In JC Hughes SJ Louw and S Sabat (eds.). *Dementia: mind, meaning and person*, pp. 287–302. Oxford University Press, Oxford.

Sabat SR (1999). Facilitating conversation with an Alzheimer's disease sufferer through the use of indirect repair. In H Hamilton (ed.). *Language and communication in old age: multidisciplinary perspectives*, pp 115–134, Garland.

Sabat SR and Harré R (1992). The construction and deconstruction of self in Alzheimer's disease. *Ageing and Society*, **12**: 443–461.

Sabat SR and Harré R (1994). The Alzheimer's disease sufferer as a semiotic subject. *Philosophy, Psychiatry, and Psychology*, **1**: 145–60.

Sabat S, Napolitano L and Fath H (2004). Barriers to the construction of a valued social identity: a case study of Alzheimer's disease. *American Journal of Alzheimer's Disease and Other Dementias*, **19**(3): 177–85.

Sacks H (1974). On the analyzability of stories by children. In R Turner (ed.). *Ethnomethodology*, pp. 216–32. Penguin, New York.

Sainfort F, Ramsey JD and Monato J (1995). Conceptual and methodological sources of variation in the measurement of nursing facility quality: an evaluation of 24 models and an empirical study. *Medical Care Research and Review*, **52**(1): 60–87.

Sampson E, Gould V, Lee D and Blanchard M (2006). Differences in care received by patients with and without dementia who died during acute hospital admission: a retrospective case note study. *Age and Ageing*, **35**, 187–9.

Sampson EL, Ritchie CE, Lai R, Raven PW and Blanchard MR (2005). A systematic review of the scientific evidence for the efficacy of a palliative care approach in advanced dementia. *International Psychogeriatrics*, **17**(1): 31–40.

Sandberg O, Gustafson Y, Brannstrom B and Bucht G (1998). Prevalence of dementia, delirium and psychiatric symptoms in various care settings for the elderly. *Scandinavian Journal of Social Medicine*, **26**(1): 56–62.

Sanders S and Corley CS (2003). Are they grieving? A qualitative analysis of examining grief in caregivers of individuals with Alzheimer's disease. *Social Work in Health Care*, **37**(3): 35–53.

Sandman L (2005). *A good death: on the value of death and dying*. Open University Press, Maidenhead.

Saunders C (1998). Quoted in 'Commitments on caring for Cancer'. In *Information Exchange*, pp. 6–7, 25 June, National Council for Hospices and Specialist Palliative Care Services, London.

Sayce L (1999). *From psychiatric patient to citizen: overcoming discrimination and stigma*. Palgrave Macmillan, London.

Sayers GM and Nesbit T (2002). Ageism in the NHS and the Human Rights Act 1998: an ethical and legal enquiry. *European Journal of Health Law*, **9**(1): 5–18.

Schag CC and Heinrich RL (1990). Development of a comprehensive quality of life measurement tool: CARES. *Oncology*, **4**(5): 135–8.

Scherder E, Oosterman J, Swaab D, Herr K, Ooms M, Ribbe M, Sergeant J, Pickering G and Benedetti F (2005). Recent developments in pain in dementia. *BMJ*, **330**(7489): 461–4.

Scheurich JJ and Bell McKenzie K (2005). Foucault's methodologies: archaeology and genealogy In NJ Denzin and YS Lincoln (eds.). *The Sage handbook of qualitative research*, 3rd edn, pp. 841–68. Sage, Thousand Oaks, CA.

Schulz R, Mendelsohn AB, Haley WE, Mahoney D, Allen RS, Zhang S, Thompson LA and Belle SH (2003). End-of-life care and the effects of bereavement on family caregivers of persons with dementia. *New England Journal of Medicine*, **349**(20): 1936–42.

Seale C (1998). *Constructing death: the sociology of dying and bereavement*. Cambridge University Press, Cambridge.

Seale CF and van des Geest S (eds.) (2004). Special issue on "Good and Bad Death" *Social Science and Median*. Vol **58**.

Seymour J (2001). *Critical moments: death and dying in intensive care*. Open University Press, Buckingham.

Seymour J, Clark D and Winslow M (2005). Pain and palliative care: the emergence of new specialities. *Journal of Pain and Symptom Management*, **29**(1): 2–13.

Shega JW, Levin A, Hougham GW, Cox-Hayley D, Luchins DJ, Hanrahan P, Stocking C and Sachs GA (2003). Palliative Excellence in Alzheimer Care Efforts (PEACE): A programme description. *Journal of Palliative Medicine*, **6**(2): 315–20.

Sheldon JH (1961). *Report of the Birmingham Regional Hospital Board on its geriatric services*. Birmingham Regional Hospital Board, Birmingham.

Simonds W and Rothman BK (1992). *Centuries of solace. Expressions of maternal grief in popular literature*. Temple University Press, Philadelphia.

Singer PA, Martin DK and Kelner M (1999). Quality end-of-life care. Patients' perspectives. *Journal of the American Medical Association*, **281**: 163–8.

Small JA (2004). Communication strategies in Alzheimer care giving; Recommended, reported and implemented. In B Vellas, LJ Fitten, B Winbard, H Feldman, M Grudman, E Giacobini (eds.). *Research and Practice in Alzheimer's Disease and Cognitive Decline*, **9**: 185–189.

Small JA, Gutman G, Makela S and Hillhouse B (2003). Effectiveness of communication strategies used by caregivers of persons with Alzheimer's disease during activities of daily living. *Journal of Speech, Language, and Hearing Research*, **46**: 353–67.

Small N (1989). *Politics and planning in the NHS*. Open University Press, Buckingham.

Small N (1993). *AIDS: the challenge*. Avebury, Aldershot.

Small N (2000). The modern hospice movement: 'bright lights sparkling' or 'a bit of heaven for the few'? In P Thompson and J Walmsley (eds.). *Oral history, health and welfare*, pp.288–308. Routledge, London.

Small N (2001). Theories of grief: a critical review. In J Hockey, J Katzs and N Small, (eds.). *Grief, mourning and death ritual*, pp. 19–48. Open University Press, Buckingham.

Small N and Rhodes P (2000). *Too ill to talk. User involvement and palliative care*. Routledge, London.

Small N, Downs M and Froggatt K (2006). Improving end-of-life care for people with dementia – the benefits of combining UK approaches to palliative care and dementia care. In BML. Meisen and GMM Jones (eds.). *Care-giving in dementia. Research and implications*, volume 4, pp. 365–92. Brunner-Routledge, London.

Smeele H (2002). *Met de Moed van een Ontdekkingsreiziger*. Servire, Utrecht.

Smith J (2005). A good death or a public one? *BMJ*, **330**: 7495.

Smith SC, Lamping DL, Banerjee S, Harwood R, Foley B, Smith P, Cook JG, Murray J, Prince M, Mann A and Knapp M (2005). Measurement of health-related quality of life for people with dementia: development of a new instrument (DEMQOL) and an evaluation of current methodology. *Health Technology Assessment*, **9**(10).

Snow AL and Shuster JL Jr (2006). Assessment and treatment of persistent pain in persons with cognitive and communicative impairment. *Journal of Clinical Psychology*, **62**(11): 1379–87.

Sorrell J (2005). Struggling to do the right thing: stories from people living with Alzheimer's disease. *Journal of Psychosocial Nursing and Mental Health Services*, **43**(7): 13–16.

Steinhardt B (1998). *Report to the Secretary of Health and Human Services: Alzheimer's disease, estimates of prevalence in the United States*. United States General Accounting Office, Washington DC.

Stokes G (2003). *Challenging behaviour in dementia: a person-centred approach*. Speechmark Publishing, Bicester.

Strauss A and Glaser B (1977). *Anguish*. Martin Robinson, London.

Stroebe MS, Hansson RO, Stroebe W and Schut H (eds) (2001). *Handbook of bereavement research: consequences, coping and care*. American Psychological Association, Washington.

Stroebe MS, Stroebe W and Hansson RO (eds) (1993). *Handbook of bereavement: theory, research and intervention*. Cambridge University Press, Cambridge.

Sudnow D (1967). *Passing on. The social organisation of dying*. Prentice-Hall, New Jersey.

Surr C (2005). Preservation of self in people with dementia living in residential care: A socio-biographical approach. *Social Science and Medicine*, **62**(7): 1720–30.

Sweeting H and Gilhooly M (1991–1992). Doctor, am I dead? A review of social death in modern societies. *Omega*, **24**(4): 251–69.

Sweeting H and Gilhooly M (1997). Dementia and the phenomenon of social death. *Sociology of Health and Illness*, **19**(1): 93–117.

Tappen RM, Williams C, Fischman S and Touhy T (1999). Persistence of self in advanced Alzheimer's disease. *Image Journal of Nursing Scholarship*, **31**(2): 121–5.

ten Have HAMJ (2004). Expanding the scope of palliative care. In RB Purtillo and HAMJ ten Have (eds.). *Ethical foundations of palliative care for Alzheimer's disease*, pp. 61–79. Johns Hopkins University Press, London.

Thunedborg K, Alerup P, Bech P and Joyce CRB (1993). Development of the repertory grid for measurement of individual quality of life in clinical trials. *International Journal of Methods in Psychiatric Research*, **3**(1): 45–56.

Tobin S (1999). *Preservation of the self in the oldest years*. Springer Publishing, New York.

Tomandl S (1991). *Coma work and palliative care: an introductory communications skill manual for supporting people living near death*. Coma Communications, Victoria, BC.

Toscani F, Borreani C, Boeri P and Miccinesi G (2003). Life at the end of life: belief about individual life after death and 'good death' models – a qualitative study. *Health and Quality of Life Outcomes*, **1**(1): 65.

Townsend P (1962). *The last refuge: a survey of residential institutions and homes for the aged in England and Wales*. Routledge and Kegan Paul, London.

Treichler PA (1992). AIDS, HIV and the cultural construction of reality. In G Herdt and S Lindenbaum (eds.). *The time of AIDS*, pp. 65–98. London, Sage.

Treloar A (2006). Hope for home: the terminal care of people with dementia at home. In *Palliative care for people with dementia. Leveson Paper Number Twelve*, pp 10–15. The Foundation of Hady Katherine Leveson, Temple Balsall.

Treloar A, Newport J and Venn-Treloar J (2005). Specialist palliative care in dementia (letter). *BMJ*, **330**(7492): 672.

Tudor-Hart J (1971). The inverse care law. *The Lancet*, 27 Feb, 405–12.

Tugwell P, Bombardier C, Buchanan WW, Goldsmith CH, Grace E and Hanna B (1987). The MACTAR Patient Preference Disability Questionnaire. *Journal of Rheumatology*, **14**(3): 446–51.

Turner K, Chye R, Agarwal G, Philip J, Skeels A and Lickiss JN (1996). Dignity in dying: a preliminary study of patients in the last three days of life. *Journal of Palliative Care*, **12**(2): 7–13.

Twigg J (2000). Carework as a form of bodywork. *Ageing and Society*, **20**(4): 389–411.

Twigg J (2004). The body, gender and age: feminist insights in social gerontology. *Journal of Ageing Studies*, **18**: 59–73.

Twigg J (2006). *The body in health and social care*. Palgrave Macmillan, London.

Twigg J and Atkin K (1994). *Carers perceived: policy and practice in informal care*. Open University Press, Milton Keynes.

United Nations General Assembly (2006). *Final report of the Ad Hoc Committee on a Comprehensive and Integral International Convention on the Protection and Promotion of the Rights and Dignity of Persons with Disabilities*. United Nations, New York. A/61/611.

Vallelly S, Evans S, Fear T and Means R (2006). *Opening doors to independence*. Housing 21, London.

Volicer L (1986). Need for hospice approach to treatment of patients with advanced progressive dementia. *Journal of American Geriatrics Society*, **34**(9): 655–8.

Volicer L, Collard A, Hurley A, Bishop C, Kern D and Karon S (1994). Impact of special care unit for patients with advanced Alzheimer's disease on patients' discomfort and costs. *Journal of the American Geriatrics Society*, **42**(6): 597–603.

Volicer L, Seltzer B, Rheame Y, Fabiszewski K, Hen L, Shapiro R and Innis P (1987). Progression of Alzheimer-type dementia in institutionalized patients: a cross-sectional study. *Journal of Applied Gerontology*, **6**: 83–94.

Walter T (1993). Sociologists never die: British sociology and death. In D Clark (ed.). *The sociology of death: theory, culture, practice*, pp. 264–95. Blackwell, Oxford.

Walter T (1994). *The revival of death*. Routledge, London.

Walter T (1996). A new model of grief: Bereavement and biography. *Mortality*, **1**(1): 7–25.

Walter T (1999). *On bereavement. The culture of grief*. Open University Press, Buckingham.

Walters G (2004). Is there such a thing as a good death? *Palliative Medicine*, **18**(5): 404–08.

Ware JE Jr (1984). Conceptualizing disease impact and treatment outcomes. *Cancer*, **53**: 2316–23.

Warnock M (2006). When to die. In *The Observer*, May 7th p. 31.

Wary B (2003). Geriatrics and palliative care: the best of both worlds. *European Journal of Palliative Care*, **10**(2 Suppl): 29–31.

Weathers L (2002–2003). Learning to let go. *Alzheimer's Society Newsletter*. December–January: 10.

Welie JVM (2004). The tendency of contemporary decision-making strategies to deny the condition of Alzheimer's disease. In RB Purtilo and HAMJ ten Have (eds.). *Ethical foundations of palliative care for Alzheimer's disease*, pp. 163–80. Johns Hopkins University Press, Baltimore.

Werner P (2006). Lay perceptions regarding the competence of persons with Alzheimer's disease. *International Journal of Geriatric Psychiatry*, **21**(7): 674.

Whitlatch C and Feinberg LF (2003). Planning for the future together in culturally diverse families: making everyday care decisions. *Alzheimer's Care Quarterly*, **4**(1): 50–61.

Whitlatch CJ, Judge KS, Zarit SH and Femia E (2006). Dyadic intervention for family caregivers and care receivers in early-stage dementia. *The Gerontologist*, **46**(5): 688–94.

Wilcock G, Bucks R S and Rockwood K (eds) (1999). *Diagnosis and management of dementia: a manual for memory disorders teams*. Oxford, Oxford University Press.

Williamson J, Stokoe IH, Gray S, Fisher M, Smith A, McGhee A and Stephenson E (1964). Old people at home: their unreported needs. *The Lancet*, **I**: 1117–20.

Wilson SA, Kovach CR and Stearns SA (1996). Hospice concepts in the care for end-stage dementia. *Geriatric Nursing*, **17**(1): 6–10.

Wittgenstein L (1953). *Philosophical investigations*. Macmillan, New York.

Woods RT (1989). *Alzheimer's disease: coping with a living death*. Souvenir Press, London.

Woods RT (2001). Discovering the person with Alzhermer's disease: Cognitive, emotional and behavioural aspects. *Ageing and Mental Health*, **5**, 57–516.

Woods RT and Britton PG (1977). Psychological approaches to the treatment of the elderly. *Age and Ageing*, **6**: 104.

Woods RT and Britton PG (1985). *Clinical psychology with the elderly*. Croom-Helm, London.

Woods RT and Clare L (eds.) (in press). *Handbook of the clinical psychology of ageing*, 2nd edn. Wiley Publishers, Chichester.

Woods RT and Holden U (1982). *Reality orientation: psychological approaches to the 'confused' elderly*. Churchill Livingstone, London.

Woods RT, Keady J and Seddon D (2007). *Involving families in care homes: a relationship-centred approach to dementia care*. Jessica Kingsley Publishers, London.

Woods, RT (1999). The person in dementia care. *Generations*, **23**: 35–39.

World Health Organization (1986). *Ottawa Charter for Health Promotion*. World Health Organization, Geneva.

World Health Organization (2002) *Palliative care*. Available at http://www.who.int/cancer/palliative/en, accessed 26 February 2007.

World Health Organization/Geriatric and Psychiatry Section of the World Psychiatric Association (1996). *Psychiatry of the elderly. A consensus statement*. World Health Organization, Geneva.

Young M and Cullen L (1996). *A good death: conversations with East Londoners*. Routledge, London.

Zarit SH (2006). The history of caregiving in dementia. In SM LoboPrabhu, VA Molinari and JW Lomax (eds.). *Supporting the caregiver in dementia: a guide for health care professionals*, pp. 3–22. The John Hopkins University Press, Baltimore.

Zarit SH and Braungart ER (2006). Elders as care receivers: autonomy in the context of frailty. In H-W Wahl, C Tesch-Romer and A Hoof (eds.). *New dynamics in old age: individual, environmental and societal perspectives*, pp. 85–104. Baywood, Amityville, NY.

Zarit SH and Gaugler JE (2006). Care by families for late stage dementia. In A Burns and B Winblad (eds.). *Severe dementia*, pp. 185–92. John Wiley and Sons, Chichester.

Zarit SH, Orr NK and Zarit JM (1985). *The hidden victims of Alzheimer's disease: families under stress*. New York University Press, New York.

Zeisel J, Silverstein NM, Hyde J, Levkoff S, Powell Lawton M and Holmes M (2003). Environmental correlates to behavioral health outcomes in alzheimer's special care units. *The Gerontologist*, **43**: 697–711.

Zimmerman S, Sloane PD, Heck E, Maslow K and Schulz R (2005). Dementia care and quality of life in assisted living and nursing homes. *The Gerontologist*, **45**(1): 5–7.

Index